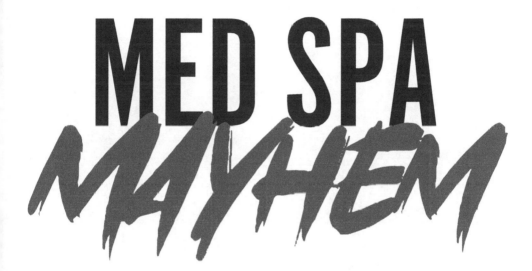

A MEMOIR + EXPOSÉ BY

DR. KATE DEE

MED SPA
MAYHEM

THE GOOD, THE BAD, AND THE UGLY
SECRETS OF THE AESTHETIC INDUSTRY

Advantage | Books

Published by Advantage Books, Charleston, South Carolina.
An imprint of Advantage Media.

ADVANTAGE is a registered trademark, and the Advantage colophon is a trademark of Advantage Media Group, Inc.

Printed in the United States of America.

10 9 8 7 6 5 4 3 2 1

ISBN: 978-1-64225-980-3 (Paperback)
ISBN: 978-1-64225-979-7 (eBook)

Library of Congress Control Number: 2024903378

Cover design by Matthew Morse.
Layout design by Megan Elger.

This publication is designed to provide accurate and authoritative information in regard to the subject matter covered. It is sold with the understanding that the publisher is not engaged in rendering legal, accounting, or other professional services. If legal advice or other expert assistance is required, the services of a competent professional person should be sought.

Advantage Books is an imprint of Advantage Media Group. Advantage Media helps busy entrepreneurs, CEOs, and leaders write and publish a book to grow their business and become the authority in their field. Advantage authors comprise an exclusive community of industry professionals, idea-makers, and thought leaders. For more information go to **advantagemedia.com**.

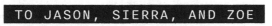
TO JASON, SIERRA, AND ZOE

CONTENTS

SECTION III: A PERSONAL AND
BUSINESS PERSPECTIVE

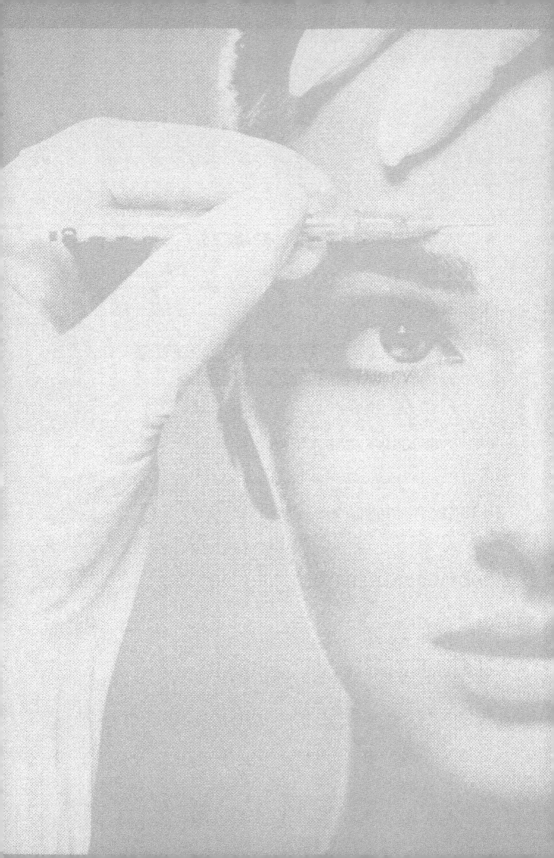

mayhem / ˈmeihem /

noun

a situation in which there is little or no order or control

confused activity or excitement, sometimes involving destructive violence

—THE CAMBRIDGE DICTIONARY

FOREWORD

Buckle up and enjoy Kate Dee's insightful and honest insider's view of med spas. As a board-certified facial plastic surgeon and aesthetic research investigator, I too have experienced many personal and professional moments described in this book. Seeing her share them in print gives a vicarious catharsis. Knowing Kate as a physician and friend, she speaks from the heart and with a conscientiousness befitting her Ivy League training. She doesn't hold back here and will keep you entertained while educating you to the pitfalls of the med spa world. I, myself, was educated by her thoughtful investigation into the legalities of running a med spa. Personally, I cannot wait for the release of the book so I can eagerly share it with my staff, colleagues, and patients. Though Kate wrote this for consumers, I believe doctors and anyone who works in the industry will devour this book. Patients and practitioners alike will learn about the chaotic world of medical aesthetics, and you will likely come away with knowledge and pearls to guide your own journey, whether or not you already participate in the med spa world. So cheers to Kate and to you for broadening your knowledge with this delightful and informative read.

—DR. YAEL HALAAS

PREFACE

I wrote *Med Spa Mayhem* to share my personal journey from a shy science geek to a so-called "beauty expert" and to uncover what I have learned along the way about the wildly dangerous practices and outright illegality of many beauty treatments, as well as to give my readers a chance to make informed decisions about aesthetic treatments. There are so many great treatments and an equal number of dangerous ones. How do you make sure you will not be another victim? My goal is that by the time you finish this book, you will know exactly what to ask and how to find the best people and treatments without risking your life or your health (or your money!).

About me: After working in medicine as a specialist in breast cancer for sixteen years, I left the hospital environment and founded Glow Medispa in 2014. I have never been a beauty consumer. I have never, in my life, worn makeup. When I was twenty-six and about to walk down the aisle (the first time), my photographer saw me and exclaimed, "Wow, Kate, you look beautiful—just the right amount of makeup!" That amount was none. I never learned to put it on. A week before, the wedding stylist who was doing my hair tried to put eye makeup on me. I was a raccoon in seconds, and she said to me, "You're such a spaz." That was the beginning and end of makeup for me.

SCIENCE GEEK BEAUTY

I have always been intimidated by the mainstream beauty industry. Walking into a fancy spa is uncomfortable, and it feels like I just don't belong there. I have no inclination to believe the impeccably made-up young girl when she tells me what she thinks will make me beautiful. I'm a science geek doctor, and I am a skeptic. When someone seems not to know how the treatment works and starts using fake science terms, I feel like I can't escape fast enough.

This does not mean I don't like to look beautiful. Absolutely I do. I just want to look like myself. Well, like myself when I was twenty-six. For a long time, I saw my twenty-six-year-old self in the mirror—in fact, I think I made it well past forty before I noticed quite a few changes had occurred while I was not paying attention. It was then that my inner geek told me to use science to approach this problem—it has always worked for me before.

In the last decade or two, there have been many dramatic scientific advances in aesthetics. Gone are the days of fat-jiggling and miracle creams. OK, there are still plenty of grifters out there, but there are many legitimate and effective treatments too. In the same way that physicists have figured out how to image the insides of your body with a giant magnet and radio waves (MRI machines don't even touch you!), scientists have figured out how to melt fat, tighten skin, and smooth wrinkles without surgery.

It has been my focus at Glow Medispa to appeal to people who believe, as I do, in natural beauty—who would be happy with a sensible approach that actually preserves healthy skin and makes you look your best as you age. My number one rule has always been safety—because nothing in aesthetics is worth any permanent harm. (It is all elective in any case.) The number two rule is effectiveness—it simply has to make sense scientifically, and it has to work. My third rule is that it has to be reasonable—both financially and in how much downtime it requires. If I look at a technology and think I wouldn't do it, I don't think my patients would either.

My goal is to reach out not only to science geeks like me but also to all those who are in a similar boat—naturally wary of anyone promising the moon but who love looking great at any age. Feeling great in your skin lends a confidence in life that cannot be overestimated. We can help you do that, with a little help from science.

I am a zebra in this industry. Look around at the med spas in your area, and you will find very few with a doctor within many miles of the place. Most are owned by a nonmedical person who is either on the beauty side or purely on the business side. They get into this business for the money—not that this is inherently wrong—but money incentivizes many decisions that are contrary to sound medical practices. Not being physicians or scientists, these spa owners often make business decisions uninformed by science. The safety and well-being of the patients are jeopardized by sheer ignorance and lack of regulation. These places hire a doctor, or sometimes mid-level providers like nurses, to be their "medical director." Oftentimes this medical director is "on paper" only and receives only a nominal payment for use of their license. We will get into the legality of these spas later. But would it surprise you to learn that most of these places are operating illegally?

This is my story and the story of the industry that has taken the world by storm, often with a lot of thunder and lightning. I hope that by the time you finish this book, you will understand how to cut through all the hype and the lies and learn what really matters and what actually works. As to who to trust, that's the hardest part of all, but I hope to give you the tools to figure out who you can truly trust with your skin.

I magine a world where the line between right and wrong is as blurred as a smudged eyeliner. Welcome to the fast-paced, glamorous, and sometimes murky world of aesthetics—a modern Wild West where ambiguity reigns supreme.

In this book, you will find the answers you've been looking for so that you can stay safe and make the right choices when you choose a medical professional to perform an aesthetic procedure.

Believe me, it could be one of the most important decisions you'll ever make.

From the traditional world of the cancer center, where medical integrity was my daily companion, I took a leap into the sparkling realm of aesthetics. What I found was a glittering facade masking a myriad of shadows. Here, amid the allure of money, the rules are not just bent, but they're often broken as well.

You might think a title like "nurse" or "doctor" guarantees legitimacy. Think again. In this glitzy arena, titles can deceive, leading the unsuspecting into a dance with danger. From back-alley Botox® to the impersonation of medical personnel, the stories I've witnessed are as jaw-dropping as they are troubling. Whistleblowing, one might assume, is the answer. Yet, in this world, the one who dares to call out the wrong often becomes the hunted. Consider the registered

nurse (RN), brimming with enthusiasm, diving headfirst into Botox®
procedures, unaware of the legal quicksand beneath her feet. As she
sinks, she searches for lifelines—sometimes in the form of online
loopholes and at other times in makeshift "solutions." The journey
from ignorance to "quasi-legality" is a complex dance, performed on
a tightrope of regulations.

But why this exposé? Why delve deep into this glittering abyss?
As a seasoned physician, I've navigated these murky waters firsthand,
from understanding all the characters in the business to the ethical
quandaries that often arise. I feel you all have the right to know. With
each chapter, we'll pull back the curtain on this industry, shining a
spotlight on the hidden corners in the hope of guiding both consumers
and practitioners to safer, more ethical shores. Join me on this eye-
opening journey as we unveil the true face of the aesthetic frontier.

ORIGIN STORY

I first knew I might not be the best fit for Big Medicine when I
hit the third year of med school. Up until then I loved everything
about my studies and introduction into the world of medicine. I
was graduated with honors and the Biology Prize from Yale with a
Bachelor of Science. I had cloned genes in the lab and written papers
on echinoids and completely geeked out on biochemistry and immu-
nology. Then at Yale Medical School, we did not have grades. It was
not just Pass/Fail, but it was also *anonymous*. I used to sign my exams
with the name Aretha Franklin or Lucille Ball (my heroes). We could
see our own scores on each test but not those of our classmates. We
were not ranked. I was motivated not by grades, but because I was
100 percent completely convinced that if I did not know *everything*,
then someone might die someday. I knew I had great grades, but my

professors and classmates did not. The only thing I had to show for my first two years, officially, were my medical boards scores. I was in the 98th percentile on the US Medical Licensing Examination (USMLE) Step 1. That gave me a false sense of security. Unfortunately, after that, medicine was no longer a meritocracy.

Third year, we started clinical rotations. That meant showing up at the hospital at five o'clock in the morning, rounding on our patients, being on the clinical team and learning as much as possible, assisting, writing notes, looking up labs, and, if you're lucky, actually being helpful to the patient's care. That's if you lucked out and got residents who liked med students and would teach as the day went by. Some residents thought of medical students as a pain in the ass or, worse, scut monkeys. Scut comprised all the menial tasks that no one in the hospital wants to do. Medical students were the scut monkeys of the hospital.

My very first rotation was in general surgery. I was assigned to a local New Haven hospital called St. Raphael's. It had its own residency program that was not quite as prestigious or well known as Yale-New Haven Hospital. I didn't know when I started that these residents did *not* like Yale medical students. Not one bit. These guys (they were all men) came from all over the country from lesser-known medical schools, and they liked to put us "Yalies" in our place. All women were referred to as "chicks"—even the one female attending surgeon they worked under. They were crass and demeaning. I was sent on scut missions daily yet otherwise ignored. Teaching was nearly nonexistent. Once I was sent in to debride (the process of removing nonliving tissue from wounds) a malodorous pressure wound on the buttocks of a paralyzed and quite belligerent patient with no instruction whatsoever—I had never even seen this done before. It was a cranky lady who needed daily debridement, and she tended to yell at anyone entering her room. It gave new meaning to a *shitty* rotation.

One day during week five out of six long weeks, we admitted a new patient for treatment of a rectal abscess. He was a very feminine gay man who was booked to a female bed before the intern did a proper exam on him. The offensive jokes went flying. My team was led by a chief resident who was a small man from Texas, and he led the charge in demeaning homophobic humor that seeped into the elevators and the cafeteria. They skipped visiting his room entirely on rounds. I would quickly run back to check on him and let him know of any updates while my team steamed ahead into the operating room (OR). I was mortified and squirming. In my head, I had told all of them off a hundred times but bit my tongue. I held it in for as long as I could. But one evening after several days of their evil mocking, I just couldn't take it any longer. I was walking to the parking garage at the same time as my chief resident and said, "I feel very uncomfortable when you make fun of [this patient]. Your jokes are out in the open in places where anyone could hear, and you don't know where his family might be." He says in his southern drawl, "Well, I come from a town in Texas where you could be beaten within an inch of your life if you're gay, and if he doesn't like it, he doesn't have to come to me as a surgeon." Without thinking, I fired back, "Well, this isn't Texas, and we don't treat people that way here. And he had no choice whether to pick you as a surgeon—he's a service patient! And you have to treat him the same as you treat everyone else." I don't remember what he said in response, if he said anything. What I remember was what happened next.

In clinical rotations, we did have grades. "Outstanding (A), Excellent (B), Very Good (C), and Good (D)." My chief resident did all he could to fail me from general surgery. A couple of weeks later, the dean of students called me into his office to show me my grade (Good) and ask me what happened. I broke down in tears. I told him all the stories. The misogyny, the insults, the scut, the homophobia. I thought my medical career was over. I had no grades from medical school but this one. Dean Gifford was very kind and reassuring. He began an investigation of St. Raphael's rotations. He interviewed every medical student who had rotated there about their experiences and found out that many of them had much worse stories than I did. In the end, he placed the entire program on probation until big changes were made, and their residents went through sensitivity training.

It was a painful lesson. I just didn't fit into the system. I watched as my classmates brownnosed their way to the top. I watched as they lied and promised every single chief resident that they were sure they would go into their specialty. That worked—the residents loved it and rewarded them with Outstandings. I couldn't do it. I managed to get Excellents and Outstandings for the rest of the year without sticking my head up anyone's rectum, but that just meant I had to know more and work harder. Those with the most scat on their noses rose the highest. Each rotation was fascinating, and I learned a ton, but nothing felt like a good fit. It felt like a crazy hierarchical toxic dystopia.

One rotation after the next, I found refuge in only one place—radiology. On every day of every rotation, we had what were called "x-ray rounds." We would make our rounds in the wards for three to four hours in the morning and invariably stop by radiology sometime midday. The radiologists seemed to have all the answers. Everything we did depended on imaging, and the radiologists would tell us what they found, what the differential diagnosis was, and, most important, what to do next. They were the puzzle solvers. They made sense. They knew so much about every disease. Plus they almost never wore scrubs!

At some point during my third year, I had developed an aversion to the big boxy cotton/polyester blend scrubs with the number 5 all over them. Someone in hospital administration had decided that if they put the ugliest number (that being the number "5") all over the blue scrubs, people would be spotted throughout New Haven as hospital-wear thieves and that this would be a deterrent to theft. It had the opposite effect. They became a fashion statement. People paired scrub tops with cute jeans and a blazer and wore them to restaurants. Except for me. I hated them. And they were not flattering.

The two radiologists I came in contact with most often were both incredibly intelligent women whom the attendings and residents all highly respected. Every day on x-ray rounds, we would meet with them, absorb their wisdom, and move on to enact their recommendations. X-ray rounds might be only twenty minutes, but I longed to stay in the department rather than return to the wards. I arranged to do a radiology elective toward the end of my third year so that I could work with Dr. Curtis and Dr. Shaw and know for sure this was my path. I was determined to follow in their footsteps. They were brilliant puzzle-solving, normal clothes-wearing women. Plus they wore great earrings. I was determined to be a brilliant puzzle-solving, gorgeous earring-wearing radiologist. Ultimately, I asked Dr. Shaw to write me a recommendation, and she warned me that radiology had become one of the most difficult specialties to get into, along with neurosurgery and dermatology. At the time I could not fathom doing anything else. It was the only place I felt at home. She said I'd have to have great grades and a top board score to get in. Armed with my 98th percentile and my dean's letter, I managed to match in my dream city, Seattle.

Internship year was one of total chaos for me. I got married and divorced and came out as gay and moved across the country to a city where I knew not a soul. I was on call every third or fourth night and did not miss a day of work. I even got regular exercise, had a social life, and made friends. Having grown up in the '70s and '80s, I was a complete *M*A*S*H* fan. I dealt with the stress like Hawkeye did (Alan Alda—another hero). Everything became a joke because if I thought about it for too long, I might just lose it. But there was no pretending to be crazy to get a weekend pass to Tokyo.

Shockingly, radiology was no haven. It was even more male dominated than most other specialties. And very conservative. I didn't know whether I could be out in my department. I didn't really know how to be out since I was so newly out to myself. I had no practice at it. The old white guys were in charge, and I wasn't sure if they would accept this new me that I had just learned to accept in myself. In the beginning, I didn't tell anyone about my life. Over time, though, it was impossible for me to keep a lid on it. I have never been able to stifle myself in this way, just as I could never lie or brownnose. I wish I could say that it made no difference, but I know this not to be true. Seattle may be a liberal town, but the world of radiology was not. The one thing I had always loved—the science—was my safe place. I took refuge in the physics of what we could do, the pathophysiology, and the manifestations of just about every disease. Radiologists study almost everything in medicine, and it was like the biggest puzzle ever made. It was a great home for a super science geek.

During my residency training, I found that it was hard to be a woman in a male-dominated field. Patients and doctors alike assumed I was a nurse or file clerk. When medical teams came for x-ray rounds, they turned to my junior male colleagues for answers because they had gray in their hair and had more gravitas and respect despite the fact I was senior and much more knowledgeable. The one area where I had a big advantage was in breast imaging. If I walked into a room with my male attending with a gray beard, I got all the questions and eye contact. These female patients trusted me. And I was a natural at interventional procedures with wires and needles. It was a great fit. Fast-forward through a top Breast Fellowship at the University of California–San Francisco (UCSF) and a sixteen-year career as a breast imaging specialist.

I fell into aesthetics by sheer accident. For sixteen years, I lived breast cancer. I performed needle procedures all day and walked women (and a few men) through their diagnoses. I loved my job. I felt like I was helping, one person at a time. One day, two colleagues whom I knew quite well came to tell me they were retiring. They were gynecology specialists who had been referring their patients to me for many years, and I had come to know them and respect them for the great care they offered their patients. I was heartbroken to see them go. They assured me that their GYN patients would be transferred to a local OB/GYN group and would still be able to see me for their breast care. But their aesthetic patients had nowhere to go.

Aesthetic patients? They told me they had been practicing aesthetic medicine for almost ten years and they loved it. They encouraged me to check it out, as it was "right up my alley." It was all needle procedures and talking to (mostly) women all day—but you make them happy! Now after sixteen years of breast cancer—making people happy sounded incredibly appealing. They invited me to follow them for a day in their clinic before they closed their office so I could see what it was all about. It was the most fun I'd had in medicine ever— with the exception of the annual ski day in my residency, where we got one day off a year to ski.

I searched for a great aesthetics course to take. That was challenging, as there are a lot of schlocky classes in the field, often taught by people who do not even have qualifications to inject. But I found one for MDs only taught by MDs. I signed up figuring that if I liked it, I would do more classes. If I didn't, at least I'd get some CME (Continuing Medical Education—all doctors must complete many hours of CME each year to maintain their license. In my state, it is fifty hours/year). The first day of this course was all on laser physics. I was in heaven. It turned out I loved all of it—Lasers, Injectables, Peels, Cosmeceuticals. It was a revelation to be able to approach beauty from a vantage point that I understood. It became demystified for me. Before then, it all seemed so superficial and filled with hype and an emphasis on the fake (lashes, boobs). Now I was learning about using science to make the skin healthier and preserve as much of your natural youth as possible.

Thus began my personal self-directed residency in aesthetic medicine. I signed up immediately for the next level course, and after that, every opportunity I could find to acquire additional training. I joined ASLMS, one of the only professional societies that would allow noncore physicians like myself to join. I bought every textbook and signed up for every hands-on training I could. I demoed every laser, every device I could get my hands on. To this day, I have continued to take advantage of every opportunity to improve my skills and make myself an expert in what I do.

HARASSMENT

In my last two years at the breast center, I was being harassed by a middle manager. When Claire (not her real name) first arrived at the hospital several years before, she was bright and helpful. She knew of me because at her previous hospital, she had worked with my ex, also a radiologist. She came by the breast center periodically and asked if there was anything she could do for us to make things run more smoothly. I thought she was the only administrator who actually cared. Over time, she befriended me and several other key people in the department. She was on her way up, rapidly displacing other managers to rise higher in the ranks of the hospital. One of the people she displaced was a woman who gave lip service to a lot of action items but never got anything done. I wasn't upset that she got the boot. I thought Claire was the kind of person who could get things done. But I should have been paying attention. Claire was one of those who got ahead in her career by destroying others.

Claire slowly extended her power across the department. She created rules to insert herself between the doctors and the techs and the administration. She stirred up discontent wherever she could. She encouraged people to write one another up and to report any and all grievances, creating an atmosphere of fear and anger throughout the department. Everyone feared for their jobs. The doctors were afraid to confront her because they were being written up too. At one point, she created a rule that no radiologist could give direct feedback to a tech. It had to go through her. Any direct feedback would be construed as harassment by the physician. Before this "rule" could be enacted, the doctors had to agree to the new policy. I went out on a limb and recommended to my group that we say no. We had to have the ability to correct technique, to optimize imaging for diagnostic quality. It wasn't harassment to ask for a different sequence on an MRI or an additional look with ultrasound. We voted her down. Unfortunately, Claire found out it was my opposition to her plan. I was her target after that.

Then there was a showdown. She was trying to fire the best (and highest paid) techs in the breast center. The techs came to me daily for help and support. I knew them to be hardworking and excellent at their jobs. They were being targeted by Claire. She wanted them out. And what Claire wanted, she got, one way or another. I stood up for the techs. They were smart and talented, they hustled to get the job done, and they truly cared about our patients. It was a war now.

Suddenly, I was being written up for unsubstantiated "crimes." I had been there for thirteen years and had not one complaint. I had the respect of the surgeons and oncologists and the love of my patients and techs. But now a series of accusations came from two people that Claire had found to be weak and could be manipulated.

Before I knew it, I was being called before the chief of surgery for these write-ups. I tried to explain the situation with Claire and the trumped-up charges, but he wasn't hearing any of it. I went to the head administrators of the hospital and tried to explain to them what I saw as an attempt at manipulative destruction. The main department and the breast center were happy and very productive "families" before Claire arrived. She was pitting people against one another, fomenting distrust and anger, and getting people fired. But in their view, this was just a catfight between "girls." I had better "own up" and admit wrongdoing and tell him my plan to fix my bad behavior, or I would be put on probation. Capitulate to this psychotic scenario or possibly lose my career. So I did exactly that. I groveled. I was left with a deep resentment that someone who was so manipulative, such a liar, so destructive and evil could rise up and take power, ruining lives and friendships and careers and go undetected, much less unpunished. It wasn't long after that I handed in my resignation. It would be another year before a similar character took over the country. (Post note: they fired Claire about a year later.)

One thing I did learn from this experience is that though I had been working there for thirteen years, I had no five-star reviews to show for it. I had nothing—no documentation of the lives I had helped or even saved. No documentation from the patients or the doctors I had been taking care of for all that time. When a restaurant has years of four- and five-star reviews, and then comes along a one-star review from a customer who thought the meal took too long, it doesn't carry much sway.

But if all you have is a one-star review from a competitor down the street, how is anyone to know which doctors have done great work and can be trusted and which cannot? It can sometimes be difficult to discern the true quality of any business or person through online reviews. There are so many fake ones out there. But a lot of us put effort into asking for them from everyone who gives us feedback.

For treatments you want to have done, always look for med spas that are not all just showing five-star reviews. These med spas will always have some four-star ones in addition to the occasional one- or two-star reviews. You can't please all of the people all of the time. But you can usually tell from the testimonials whether a med spa and its people are serving their clients well. If only the hospital systems had a legitimate way of assessing the quality of the medical care being provided. It's not about the money. It's not even how much the patients loved their bedside nurse. It is about the whole experience and the outcomes. Hospitals are just way behind the rest of the economy when it comes to user experience and worker satisfaction.

Starting my own business meant I could focus all of my energy on both of those things. All of our business decisions must make business and medical sense and improve the happiness of both our patients and our staff. As you read on, keep in mind that most of the med spas you're reading about are each their own microcosm, each an experiment in healthcare. As you'll see, no one is policing them. This book will help you understand all the aspects of the crazy world of med spas and hopefully avoid the mayhem.

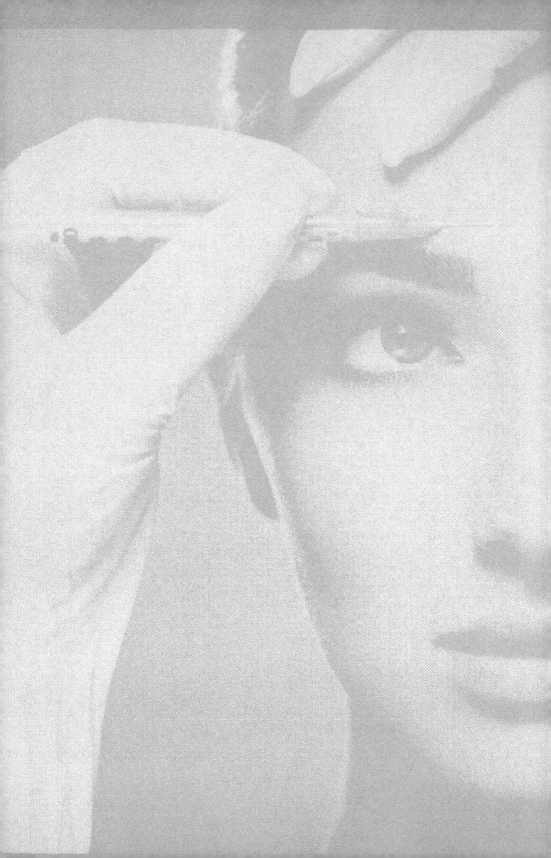

SECTION 1

THE INTRIGUING WORLD OF AESTHETICS AND ITS PLAYERS

Diving into the beauty world? It's not all glitz and glam. In this chapter, we're lifting the lid on some shady industry secrets. With stories from the inside and some real-deal science, we'll help you spot the genuine from the fake. By the end, you'll know how to get that glow safely. Ready to see the real side of beauty? Let's dive in!

CHAPTER 1

THE AESTHETICS REVOLUTION

A forty-seven-year-old mother of four walked into a med spa in Wortham, Texas, to have a routine IV vitamin infusion. She was dead minutes later. The "licensed professional" who killed her did not have any license, and the "medical director" lived and worked full-time over one hundred miles away in Dallas.

A healthy forty-nine-year-old woman who wanted to improve her jowls and sagging skin endures an excruciating series of injections resulting in disfigurement, after seeing a nurse practitioner (NP) for treatment in a medical spa in Seattle.

Linda Evangelista, a celebrity supermodel in the 1990s, sues the maker of CoolSculpting® in 2021, citing body disfigurement, later settling in 2022 for $50 million.

The story of the aesthetics industry is one of success, beauty, and lots of money. It is also one of deception, disfigurement, and death. In this book, you will learn all the ways the med spa industry shines, along with how medical aesthetics can be dark, unethical, and criminal. Meet the characters and companies behind the curtain, and find out how to get the best treatments and avoid the pitfalls.

THE TURF BATTLE

The aesthetics economy exploded from a $10 billion industry in 2019 to an eye-popping $99.1 billion in 2021, just two years later. It is expected to expand at a compound annual rate of 14.5 percent through 2030. This tremendous influx of dollars has spurred the most vicious and contentious battles in medicine. Everyone wants a piece of the action. In this chapter, I'll explain the players and their role in the battle, and will try to give you a basis for putting what each of them says into context.

THE BIRTH OF THE AESTHETICS INDUSTRY

It helps to start at the beginning to see how this contest started. The field of aesthetic medicine is inextricably linked to the creation and rise of Botox® and Restylane® for cosmetic use. The bacterium *Clostridium botulinum* that causes botulism was first isolated in Belgium in the 1800s, but the toxin itself wasn't purified in the lab until the 1920s in the United States. The toxin was actually weaponized by the US military and their scientists during World War II, and after the war was over, the toxin was provided to academic scientists for study. Eventually, an ophthalmologist named Alan B. Scott perfected the techniques for manufacturing the toxin and got the Food and Drug Administration's (FDA) approval to use it for investigative use in the 1970s. He injected the first patient with strabismus (the official term for being cross-eyed) in 1977. He called his toxin Oculinum, a drug that could align the eye. He did well with the product until the insurance companies shut him down—they would not provide product liability insurance. Botulism wasn't something they were willing to insure. Botulinum toxin became very scarce very quickly until Allergan came along and bought the rights to the toxin, dubbing it "Botox®" for the first time. They quickly trademarked the name.

Based on the investigations of hundreds of scientists that had already been done using Dr. Scott's toxin, Allergan was able to obtain the first official approval from the FDA for clinical use to treating muscle spasm in 1989. It was then used for various different kinds of medical conditions involving overactive muscles. It was a godsend for these patients. If you have never heard of hemifacial spasm, imagine if half of your face were curled up into a twisted rope all the time because of spasm of the muscles of your face. It can be quite disfiguring. When injected with Botox®, the muscles relax and the face returns to a normal appearance at rest. The downside is that you can't move them, so when you smile, the other side of your face can do that, but the treated side remains placid. You can imagine that doctors over the years tried to treat with just the right amount to relax the spasm, but tried to leave people with some movement, so that they can still smile and look relatively normal. In that first decade of experimentation with Botox®, doctors found that they could fairly precisely treat various muscle groups to treat a variety of muscular spasm problems. They also noticed what we all know now—that wrinkles disappeared as well.

In 2002, Allergan obtained the first FDA approval for Botox® to treat glabellar lines (the 11's between the eyebrows). At that time, they created the name "Botox Cosmetic®" for the name of the same toxin for use to treat facial wrinkles, while plain "Botox®" was still used for medical purposes. The difference is important mostly because "Botox®" is reimbursable by insurance companies for medical uses (muscle spasm, migraines), whereas Botox Cosmetic® is used for aesthetics only.

Dysport® is a similar neurotoxin owned by the company Galderma, based in Switzerland. Dysport® was approved for use in Europe in 1990, just one year after Botox® in the United States, and was eventually FDA-approved for use in the United States in 2009. Botox® and Dysport® are by far the most common toxins used in the United States today. Xeomin® is another toxin offered by the company Merz, based in Germany. It was approved for use in Europe in 2007 and was then FDA-approved for cosmetic use in the United States in 2011. The newer toxins on the market in the United States, Daxxify Jeuveau® and Daxxify®, were FDA-approved in 2019 and 2022, respectively. Throughout this book, these products are collectively referred to as "toxin" or "neurotoxin."

The aesthetics industry is still in its infancy. I would mark the birth of the industry as the date of the first approval of Botox Cosmetic® in 2002. The very next year, in 2003, Restylane® became the very first dermal filler made from hyaluronic acid (what the vast majority of fillers are made from now) to be FDA-approved for cosmetic use. Suddenly in the early 2000s, there were injectable tools to treat lines and wrinkles of the face, and they were not covered by insurance. People who wanted to improve their skin and look younger with these new tools had to pay cold hard cash. And they needed access to a doctor to have the treatments. This was something that most doctors had no experience with. Doctors in Big Medicine are usually completely separate from billing and insurance. Most do not even know the cost of the treatments and procedures they recommend for their patients.

PLASTIC SURGEONS

There was one exception to this: plastic surgeons. Plastic surgery is divided into two main segments: cosmetic and reconstructive. Reconstructive surgery is needed after an injury has occurred, and the body part must be rebuilt. For example, a car accident causing facial injury or breast reconstruction following breast cancer surgery. Cosmetic surgery, on the other hand, is entirely elective and is not covered by insurance. Plastic surgeons have traditionally specialized mostly in one or the other, but any plastic surgeon who performs cosmetic surgery does so for cash. People pay out of pocket because they truly desire the change that surgery offers. Plastic surgeons have the longest history of being in a cash business, and they had many years of experience in the space before Toxin and Filler showed up. And this was a perfect fit, since they were already in the cosmetic surgery business.

The only glitch was that surgeons do one very lucrative thing—surgery. They are really good at it. Plastic surgeons are incredibly well trained. They have to undergo five years of general surgery residency and then two more years of plastic surgery training. Then many will do a fellowship after that. When you include medical school, that's at least twelve years of training before they even get their first job. The talent and skill they have are maximally put to use doing surgery.

When injectables first arose, plastic surgeons around the country learned how to inject the new toxins and fillers and trained their nurses and PAs to do the injections. Surgeons spent their time performing the much more lucrative surgical procedures, and their mid-level employees did the injections. Over time, more and more plastic surgeons opened aesthetic practices, often entirely separate from their surgical practice, offering injectables and laser treatments.

These aesthetic procedures complemented the surgical work they were doing, and in many ways, they felt they owned the space.

DERMATOLOGISTS

At the same time this was happening, dermatologists were also learning about injectables and lasers. Dermatologists are specialists in the skin. Unlike plastics though, the vast majority of dermatologists specialize in medical dermatology and relatively few in cosmetic derm. Traditionally, those going into a cosmetic practice were often treated as second-class citizens by the larger medical dermatology community. And those dermatologists who practiced "cosmetic surgery" were especially shunned, not only by their fellow derms but especially by the plastic surgeons. Plastic surgeons who train all those years to do plastics absolutely hated that derms came along (just three years of dermatology residency and a year of cosmetic fellowship) to take some of their cash-paying patients away. And they weren't even surgeons! Hence the first of the turf battles: the plastics versus the derms.

The medical dermatologists treat all kinds of skin conditions, rashes, and skin cancer. Although some did, most dermatology residencies did not train doctors in cosmetic derm. When toxins and fillers came along, dermatologists had to learn how to use them on the job. Like the plastic surgeons, they also trained their nurses and PAs in lasers and injectables. Just as their surgical counterparts did, they started to develop separate cosmetics practices run by nurses and PAs within their medical dermatology practices.

So here we are in the late aughts, with the derms and the plastics battling it out for these new dollars in this new industry. Enter the entrepreneurs and the noncore MDs.

ENTREPRENEURS

The next team in the battle were the businesspeople who were watching a new industry skyrocket, and they wanted to get a piece of it. These investors founded a new creation called the medical spa. They hired the same mid-level practitioners from the plastic surgeons and dermatologists and often paid them a little more money to work in a freestanding aesthetics clinic that offered just cosmetic products and services in a more spa-like setting. They were the first to offer spa treatments like facials and massage and medical treatments like laser hair removal and Botox® under one lovely roof. The medical spa was all about customer experience, and it took these procedures out of the sterile medical office setting.

These businesspeople could not technically own a medical practice. We will discuss the laws and legality of the medical aesthetics industry in later chapters. For now, think about this essential tenet of the law in most states: only a doctor can practice medicine or own a medical practice. How do businesspeople get around that? They hire a "medical director" for the spa. Medical directors are supposed to run the medical practice and supervise the mid-levels, and all of the medicine is done under their license. Medical spas must have a medical director to buy Botox® and other medical supplies and equipment. Businesspeople running a medical spa must have a medical director on staff. More on this in chapter 10.

Dermatologists and plastic surgeons, the core specialists, absolutely hated the new medical spas that were starting to pop up around the country. They were stealing their injectors. And their patients. And their money. And they were imposters! They are not plastic surgeons or dermatologists. Just nurses! Though the core doctors were indignant, it was a little hard to defend their own practices, since many of them did not actually inject or perform any of the laser treatments themselves. They had created this army of mid-levels for these tasks. And though they wanted to own them, they couldn't keep them siloed for long.

The businesspeople had stolen their idea and made it nicer and more comfortable. If they did a great job, why would anyone go back to the core doctors? Especially if the prices were lower in spas? Well, that all depended on how great the medical spa turned out to be. If a patient found a wonderful injector in a lovely spa, they would not go back. But these spas are all over the map in terms of quality and experience. Some would become resounding successes. Others would flounder.

NONCORE DOCTORS

Enter the wary emergency room (ER) doc. Or OB/GYN. Or internist. Or radiologist, like me. There are a lot of great doctors out there. We all have different talents, but we all have two things in common—we went to medical school, and we know how to practice medicine. Some of us were born with a needle in our hand (I was in fact twenty-two the first time I wielded a needle, but it feels like I was born to do it). Doctors may have come to aesthetics in a very directed way or have just stumbled into it as I did. But I can tell you that if you do these procedures all day every day, you get pretty good at it. That's why our nurses and PAs are so great—they are practicing the art of aesthetics every day.

Many core doctors are simply livid that a noncore, such as myself, would enter into the aesthetics world. I had no idea about this until I was shunned by one of my best friends from medical school. I had just started my business and was on the East Coast visiting my family.

I arranged to have dinner with this friend who had trained at a very prestigious dermatology program. When I told her my origin story (it's all in the preface), I had hoped she would be supportive of my new endeavor. I had thought that she knew me well, so even if she had skepticism about others in the industry, she knew I was smart and sincere and that I deeply cared about my patients. I thought she would think that if it could be done well, I would be the one to do it. Instead, she called me a "Botox®-Slinger" and told me off. She has not spoken to me since.

Why do dermatologists believe that their RN should inject Botox® but not an experienced MD? Especially when they themselves may not do any injecting at all or do it themselves only part-time? Dermatologists are the experts in the skin. I believe they feel that they are the only people who should be able to supervise aesthetic injectors and are the only people who should be managing anything to do with the skin. I wholeheartedly agree that there is no other expert to turn to for any rash, skin lesion, or skin disease. I have never pretended to be anything other than what I am—a breast cancer expert turned full-time medical aesthetics physician. If a patient wants to ask a dermatologic question, I always refer them to my favorite dermatologists for consultation. When I see a suspicious lesion, I tell them to go get it checked out. Medical spas do not offer dermatology, nor should they. But we do an amazing job of skin care and treatments to keep your skin healthy and looking its best. I asked my friend, "How much cosmetic dermatology did you do in residency?" Her answer, and the answer for any dermatologist who is my age, is *zero*. We did our residencies before this stuff was born. They learned it on the job as we did.

Interestingly, most dermatologists who do practice some cosmetic derm do so as the minority of their practice. Most are busy treating skin diseases and cancer, most of the time. As a consequence, even if they do injections themselves, they are not doing it every day, all day. Who has more experience after a few years?

This is not to say that all noncore doctors in the field are so fantastic. The truth is, if you give up your traditional Big Medicine practice to do aesthetics full-time, the market will determine your success. If you're good, people will love you, because you're a real doctor and you're there every day, you answer questions, and you know what you're doing.

THE MID-LEVELS

But wait! There's more! Now that we have created all these mid-level providers who have the skills to inject, they too want in on the action. Why should they do all the work and the business owner make all the money? If they are feeding the business such a lucrative source of income, shouldn't they be making more money? The nurses and PAs want their fair share.

With a few exceptions (see the "What Is Legal" section in chapter 10), almost all states do not allow nurses or PAs to practice on their own. But just as the businesspeople can hire a medical director, so can a nurse or PA. There are lots of medical spas owned by nurses and PAs, some set up legally, but many not so much. There has been a huge surge in mid-level injectors getting training in a dermatology office or plastic surgery practice or medical spa and taking their newfound skill and going out on their own. Guess what—*all* the doctors—cores and noncores alike—just hate this. They provide the training, marketing, and their own patients and most importantly, their liability and their license. The newly trained injector develops a following and wants to take his/her skills and patients with them. And often, they're doing it illegally!

I have been warned by innumerable doctors in aesthetics—*do not* train a new injector, especially not an NP. In my state, Washington, NPs can practice independently and can legally own a medical practice. I was told I was nuts to train a brand-new NP to do what I do. "She will leave you. It is inevitable." This is true, and it happened. In my mind, if I offer a great income and lifestyle and treat my employees with respect and fairness, they will stick around. The business side of the spa is super-hard work, and most people don't realize it until they're trying to do it.

I have personally trained one NP and one PA to be aesthetic providers. I have also hired NPs and PAs who were already trained elsewhere. We work as a team, with respect and collegiality. When it comes to medicine, it is my practice, and the buck stops here. They know I am here to consult with and respond to any question or concern. And they allow the spa to function when I am working on payroll or writing a book.

And yes, two NPs who worked for me took off on their own. In many states, this would be illegal but not in Washington. I don't begrudge them their lives or practices. If you have what it takes to make this business work, you will be successful. For every person who tries, there are more who fail. The business of aesthetics is as cutthroat as any, and anyone you speak to will tell you their stories. If you have the time, money, and risk tolerance, you may very well succeed.

I am an active participant in several online forums (fora, for fellow Latin scholars) with other aesthetics physicians, and there are frequent pileups on the mid-levels. I think it is not deserved. We are all individuals with our strengths and weaknesses, and we are all human. Some people will simply behave badly. So whether a core dermatologist, plastic surgeon, noncore physician, or a mid-level provider, you will find greatness and evil among them all. Whom to trust? You will have to get to know your specific person, talk to them, and see whether what they say makes sense. I hope that the following chapters in this book will serve as a guide on how to do that.

AESTHETICIANS, MEDICAL ASSISTANTS, DENTISTS, CHIROPRACTORS, AND NATUROPATHS

This discussion would not be complete without mentioning the plethora of other providers who are flying into and out of the aesthetics space. There are so many different entry points. Some, such as dentists, are already near the face with a needle—so why not? It is legal in many states for dentists to inject Botox® around the mouth. However, they cannot practice medicine—only dentistry. So they can't legally move to the rest of the body or manage other medical providers.

Aestheticians go to school to advise on skin care and perform facials and peels. Some states allow them to become laser technicians as well, with a higher-level "master aesthetician" licensure. However, aestheticians do not study medicine or nursing. They are not certified to handle blood or use needles. They are not trained in sterile technique. Until you have had an OR nurse yell at you to re-scrub from scratch for lowering your hands 1 centimeter, you will never really understand what it means to practice sterile technique. In my opinion, aestheticians should not be performing needle procedures. But you will find in some places, even aestheticians are injecting Botox® and fillers.

Medical assistants in most states have no licensure at all. Medical assistants are hired and trained by a clinic to help support the nurses and doctors. Some are trained as phlebotomists and can draw blood for lab use. Shockingly, some medical assistants are out there performing PRP (platelet-rich plasma) procedures and even injecting Botox®, despite their lack of licensure.

There are numerous other providers who have ventured into medical aesthetics as well. The laws guiding whether these practitioners can practice at all, much less what they are allowed to do, are well beyond the scope of this book. For the most part, these illegal practitioners are outside the system, with no oversight and no malpractice insurance. Most doctors cringe at the idea of nonmedical providers practicing medicine. The legal structure of a medical spa is discussed at length in chapter 10. There is a lot of disagreement and disparagement among the various players listed in this chapter about how medical aesthetics should be practiced, where, and by whom. The turf battle is real.

Keep in mind the forty-seven-year-old, killed by a nonlicensed provider in Texas in 2023. It matters who is doing your injections.

KEY TAKEAWAYS

FROM THIS CHAPTER

1. Research and verify the credentials of any aesthetic professional before undergoing a procedure.
2. Stay informed about any potential risks associated with treatments.
3. Check medspamayhem.com for updates.

CHAPTER 2

THE LEARNING CURVE

N avigating the medical world can be daunting, especially when faced with a myriad of credentials and certifications. Who is qualified to do what, and why? What is the required medical training background for giving Botox® or any other procedure? The success of your procedure and possibly your life depends on it.

HOW ARE DOCTORS TRAINED AND WHAT IS BOARD CERTIFICATION?

MEDICAL SCHOOL

First, you have to be accepted to a medical school. Premed requirements that you must complete in college are extensive, including full-year classes in calculus, biology, physics, inorganic chemistry, and everyone's hated organic chemistry. And English! If you have solid As in college, and you manage high scores on the MCAT (the SAT for med school), you might get into a med school. It is not easy: the overall chances of getting into a medical school are about 7 percent. One of my friends has a daughter who went through the application process in 2022. She had all As at Yale. She applied to twenty-five medical schools and got into three and wait-listed at one.

After four years of medical school, if you complete the requirements, you receive a medical doctor degree or MD. However, this does not mean you know how to practice medicine. You learn that in residency. If you haven't completed a residency, you are extremely unlikely to get a job practicing medicine in the United States.

MEDICAL BOARDS

In order to practice medicine in the United States, you must pass a series of three written tests called the USMLE, or United States Medical Licensing Exam. The first two exams are given in medical school. The third is taken during the first year of training.

RESIDENCY AND FELLOWSHIP

After med school, almost all doctors in the United States train in a residency. These are additional years of hands-on training in a specialty. This ranges from three years (e.g., family practice) to seven years (e.g., plastic surgery). Fellowship is further training after residency in a subspecialty, which is usually one to three more years.

This means that in order to practice medicine in the United States, your doctor went to college for four years and then completed anywhere from seven to thirteen years of additional education and training. That's up to seventeen years from start to finish!

WHAT IS BOARD CERTIFICATION?

The American Board of Medical Specialties (ABMS[1]) requires all of this training and multiple tests in order to qualify as board certified. Just because you completed a residency does not mean you are board certified. For that you have to pass all the tests. In the United States, it is really hard to get a job as a doctor if you are not board certified.

I am board certified in diagnostic radiology. After four years of med school, I completed one year of internal medicine internship, four years of radiology residency, and one year of subspecialty fellowship training in breast imaging. That meant I entered med school in 1990 and emerged in 2000 from my fellowship as a fully trained breast cancer expert. I got my very first job at age thirty-two. I missed the '90s! The entire decade! Just ask me anything about the '90s—I probably don't know it. When my kids started school at the same school where Eddie Vedder's kids went, I asked, "Who's that?" I swear—a decade of my life, pfffft.

What does it mean when doctors list that they are "double board certified"? If that is really true, it means they completed *two* residencies and passed the board exams for both! Wow, that would take a long time. There are definitely doctors who have done this but not many.

FAKE BOARD CERTIFICATION

Beware of people falsely claiming to be board certified. If you see a credential that says "double board certified" in any of the following categories, these are not recognized by the ABMS:

- integrative medicine
- antiaging medicine

---

1   https://www.abms.org/.

- aesthetic medicine

- cosmetic medicine

- regenerative medicine

- functional medicine

For example, Dr. Anna is a board certified OB/GYN who calls herself "triple board certified" in gynecology and obstetrics, integrative medicine, and antiaging and regenerative medicine. Just so you know, the OB/GYN is legit—and that is a ton of training and true board certification. But the others are training courses, like many of us have taken. There is no legitimate board certification in aesthetic medicine. It doesn't exist.

And Dr. Tami did not complete a residency. She is not board certified in any specialty. But she states she is "Double Board Certified in Aesthetic Medicine and Anti-aging Medicine." How can she say that? Because no one stops her from labeling herself that way. However, she has been sued by the Washington State attorney general for fraud. We'll see more about her later.

There are private organizations that have called themselves "boards" that provide training in these topics, but these training courses are counted in days, not years. For example, the American Academy of Aesthetic Medicine (AAAM) is an MD-run organization that offers a basic course for three days and an advanced course for five days. I took both when I first started on this journey. Then you can pay a few thousand dollars to take the "board" exam, and they will dub you "board certified." However, this is not recognized by the ABMS and clearly does not compare to the many years of training that true board certification entails. In fact, this type of thing is an affront to all the docs who truly dedicated their lives to learning how to practice medicine. Saying you are "double board certified" on your website or book cover does not make it true. The ABMS has a link where you can look up any physician's board certification. It is very handy.[2]

TRAINING FOR NURSES

Most nurses are Registered Nurses or RNs. Many RNs go to nursing school and get a bachelor of nursing degree, which is a college degree. However, many others become RNs after completing an associate's degree in nursing and then passing a national exam. There is no further training for RNs. Most nurses have two to four years of college.

WHAT CAN RNs DO?

What does an RN do? A good description is on the Regis College[3] web page:

Registered nurses play an important role within the healthcare community. While their exact role and responsibilities can vary significantly depending on the size of their team and the environment in which they work (for example, in a hospital, doctor's office, school, etc.), they typically include the following:

- Observing patients and conducting assessments
- Recording patient medical information and symptoms
- Updating patient files as appropriate
- Creating a patient care plan with the broader medical team

---

2   ABMS, "Verify certification," https://www.abms.org/board-certification/
     verify-certification/.

3   Regis College, "How to become a registered nurse (RN): three key steps," https://
     www.regiscollege.edu/blog/nursing/how-to-become-a-registered-nurse.

- Administering treatments and medications

- Performing care of wounds

- Collecting blood, urine, stool, and other samples for lab work

- Educating patients and their families throughout the course of treatment

Can RNs make medical decisions? No. Can they practice on their own? No. Can they own a medical practice? No (in almost every state). But sometimes they do in spite of this. That doesn't make it legal.

TRAINING REQUIREMENTS FOR NURSE PRACTITIONERS

To become an NP, one must be an RN, hold a bachelor of science in nursing (BSN), complete an NP-focused graduate master's or doctoral nursing program, and successfully pass a national NP board certification exam. Most NP programs take two years. In Washington State, NPs have the ability to practice independently. In order to get licensed, nurses have to graduate from an approved nurse practitioner program and have an active RN license. The only additional requirements are HIV/AIDS training and a personal statement. Hours of clinical experience are only required to reactivate an expired license. Thus, most NPs have a two-year master's degree. There is no residency.

ARE SOME NURSES DOCTORS?

What about nurses who get a doctorate? Some NPs get a doctorate in nursing. Do you call them doctors? Well, yes, technically, just as a doctor of economics is also a doctor. But don't be misled. There are a lot of them, but they not only do not have an MD, they also have not trained in a residency and certainly are *not* board certified. And on top of that, there are online-only nursing schools that have popped up offering Doctor of Nursing Practice degrees. Always ask who works at the spa, what are their credentials, and then look them up. You can look up any doctor on the ABMS website,[4] and find out if they are really board certified. In some states, it is illegal to call yourself a doctor when you are not—and in California, an NP (who had a doctorate and called herself a doctor) was charged with violating California's Business and Professions Code because of unfair business practices and false advertising. But in many states, NPs call themselves doctors without repercussions. It is up to you to find out who you're dealing with.

FAKE NURSES

In 2023, a scandal broke[5] where thousands of nurses were found to have purchased fake nursing degrees online. These nurses were working all over the United States, and they are still being weeded out of the system. Though nursing licenses are governed by state nursing boards, this website sponsored by the National Council of State Boards of Nursing[6] allows easy lookup of nurses to confirm their license status.

---

4   https://www.abms.org/.

5   Li Cohen, "More than 7,600 fake nursing diplomas issued in Florida in alleged wire fraud scheme," January 27, 2023, https://www.cbsnews.com/news/fake-nursing-diplomas-issued-florida-alleged-wire-fraud-scheme-justice-department/.

6   https://www.nursys.com/.

KEY TAKEAWAYS

FROM THIS CHAPTER

1. Medical Mastery Takes Time: Becoming a fully trained doctor can require up to seventeen years of education and hands-on training.

2. Board Certification Is a Gold Standard: Always verify a doctor's claims of board certification through trusted sources. Don't believe anyone claiming to be double or triple board certified without looking them up!

3. Be Informed about Medical Credentials: Not all "doctors" are MDs. Ensure you understand the qualifications of any medical professional you consult.

4. Nurses are important members of the medical team. Nursing degrees take two to four years and have no residency or post-degree training. Registered Nurses are not legally allowed to practice independently.

CHAPTER 3

NAVIGATING THE AESTHETIC LANDSCAPE

n this chapter, I'll describe why aesthetic medicine is so different from traditional medicine and why much of what we do is "scientific" but not proven. Then I'll describe just how hard it is to find the right expert provider, even if you are an expert yourself.

WHY WE HAVE LITTLE HARD DATA IN AESTHETICS

In the United States, healthcare is close to a $4 trillion industry. According to the Centers for Medicare and Medicaid (CMS), US healthcare spending reached $3.5 trillion in 2017 or $10,739 per person. As a share of the nation's gross domestic product, health spending accounted for 17.9 percent. That's a giant pot of money, and there are a lot of people vying to grab a chunk of it. That's what spurs clinical trials—the drive to prove a treatment works for a new indication means that CMS will cover it and insurance companies will follow suit. Money drives innovation, and if a new study can prove a new treatment is worth it, there is a lot of profit to be generated.

This is not how it works in aesthetics, where there are no insurers and no government payors. In medical aesthetics, every treatment is elective and cash-pay. You don't need to convince the government or insurance companies to pay for a service. You need to convince the consumer. This proves to be a far easier task, as long as you have enough advertising dollars. Let that sink in: no one is in charge of deciding whether a treatment is effective—except the consumer. You have to trust that the person selling you the service is telling you the full truth.

When a new medical device is invented, it needs to be either "approved" or "cleared" by the FDA. Once the FDA says it can be used in the United States, *doctors can use it for any indication. All they need to do is sell it to consumers. This is called Off-Label Use.*

There are two big concepts in the previous paragraph.

1. *FDA Approval versus FDA Clearance*: Most doctors don't even know that there is a difference. When a new type of device is invented and there is nothing like it that exists already, it must undergo fairly extensive and costly testing and research to prove that it reliably accomplishes a goal and is safe. The company that makes that device has to fund those studies and submit to a complex approval process. This is a pricey endeavor. However, if there is already a drug or device that has been FDA approved, and you invent a new device that is *similar to the already-approved one*, then there is a quicker, less expensive route with the FDA called 510(k) clearance. This process requires no clinical trials or much oversight. All you need to do is prove that your device or drug is "substan-tially equivalent" to the already-approved one. Most drugs

and devices sold in the US market have FDA clearance, not approval. Many devices that have FDA clearance are being sold as "new technology" even though they are not.

2. *Off-Label Use*: The second concept in that paragraph is about what you are allowed to do with that FDA seal of approval. Companies can *market* a device for only the indication that the device was originally approved or cleared. However, they can be *used* for any indication that the doctor deems appropriate. When a doctor uses a device for a purpose other than that for which it was FDA approved, it is called "Off-Label Use" of that device.

To pay for any Off-Label Procedure, unlike regular medical service like a Pap smear, there is no CMS or insurance company blocking the way. If people want to pay for it, they can and will. So doctors can use any FDA-approved or FDA-cleared device in whatever manner they like. The consumption is not linked to randomized controlled trials. Because of this, these studies never get done. Once a device passes the FDA, there are no more studies. The money it would take to get clearance for a new indication isn't worth it to the companies because it can be sold for that indication without clearance. So it just doesn't happen.

That's really a shame. Doctors like me really want that information, but we do not have the money or resources to conduct our own trials. What ends up happening is that we learn through colleagues that a treatment works by anecdotal stories, and we try it ourselves. When we find that it works for us, we keep doing it. When we find it doesn't, we drop it. But controlled trials are simply not available.

Finding the right expert in the realm of aesthetics and cosmetic treatments is crucial to your health! The consequences of trusting your face or body to an inexperienced or ill-informed practitioner can be dire, as evidenced by the horrific tales of patients who suffered from ill-advised or badly delivered treatments. This chapter delves into the challenges of distinguishing a genuine expert from a pretender, the pitfalls of falling for surface-level charm, and my own behind-the-scenes journey of assembling a team that resonates with the vision and ethos of a top-tier medical spa. Whether you're seeking treatments or looking to venture into this industry, this chapter offers insights and cautions that are invaluable.

FINDING THE RIGHT EXPERT

UNDER-EYE SAUSAGES AND SCARRING

One patient described to me her utter fear of fillers after a bad experience elsewhere. She said that a nurse injected six syringes of Voluma® in her tear troughs (under eye area). I really doubted that this could be true. First, Voluma® is not made for the tear trough. As a matter of fact, it would be one of the last fillers you might choose for that area. But also, six? That's crazy. We typically use one. Maybe two sometimes if the area really needs it. I said it must have looked like she had balloons under her eyes. She said sausages. Full-sized breakfast links. She described the nightmare of multiple sessions trying to dissolve it, but that she still had residual lumps, and she would never ever have filler again. I couldn't blame her. My only thought was, "Who in their right mind would even do that? What were they thinking?" The only conclusion is that this person had no idea what they were doing. That's why it's so important to make sure you're receiving treatment from a qualified clinician.

Another patient told me she had two syringes of Radiesse® placed in her tear troughs. Radiesse®? Never! Really? Radiesse® is an older filler that is made of calcium (yes—that's what bones are made of). It is way too firm to place in this sensitive area—and by the way is also *not* dissolvable. I don't know anyone who would even think of injecting this into the under-eye area. But someone did. This patient had a severe reaction to it. She described a bad allergic-type reaction, and her under-eye area lit up like it was on fire. She went to a dermatologist to treat it, but they had never seen this before either. She said it took seven to eight years before it was less noticeable, but she has persistent scarring. She is also someone who will never have filler again.

Let's next look at how hard it is to find the right expert. If it is hard for me, how will you do it?

A NEEDLE IN A HAYSTACK

There are many things they don't teach you in medical school. There are no business classes, no mention of money or costs of procedures, and especially no lessons in managing employees. I have always been somewhat of an empath, and I used to think I was a great judge of character. I had no clue how hard it would be hiring and managing people. Finding excellent people who are smart, expert, and kind is like finding a needle in a haystack. Mostly, I have been extremely lucky. When I was just starting out and planning to open my spa, I had people send me their résumés from all over. They heard about me somehow, and they wanted to be a part of it. I have had a fair amount of stability in my staff, but the risk one takes in hiring any new person is astronomical. How have I put together my team? It has been a tough lesson, trying to find the rose among thorns. I have a fantastic team now, but it has been a journey and a steep learning curve. Here are a few who did not work out.

Maureen

Before I even opened my spa, I was approached by a local aesthetician. Maureen (not her real name) had her own business mainly waxing in a shed in her backyard but had recently gotten training and certification as a master aesthetician. In Washington, that license allows you to perform laser treatments and work under a doctor and generally make more money. If she worked for me, she would be able to do medical treatments like laser and medical-grade peels. Ultimately, she would be able to make more money than she could waxing ladies' mustaches in her backyard.

She was all in. Until she wasn't. At first she wanted to work six days/week! Then five. Then four. Then when we were within a few weeks of opening our doors, it became three days/week. She had surmised that we would be collecting payments and reporting taxes and that she would no longer be pocketing the entire amount as cash. Once we opened, she started to block her schedule for part of the day and run home to wax clients there and then return to see medical patients. One day, I saw her collecting a cash payment right into her pocket rather than into the cash drawer. Maureen glanced up at me and realized I had seen this, and she went to the till and added the cash.

After five weeks, she walked off the job in the middle of the day. Within three months, our master aestheticians were making twice what they could on their own. This was my first lesson in managing employees and my first blessing. Anyone who would walk off the job midday was not someone you'd want on your team.

Ditzy

Ditzy worked at Glow for exactly a year. We became very busy in just a few months. She performed medical facials, microneedling, intense pulsed light (IPL), and body sculpting. She and the two other master aestheticians worked well together and, I thought, had a great camaraderie. One day she got a very bad review on Yelp. I called the patient immediately, and it turns out the patient was an aesthetician herself. She informed me that the facial she had made no sense. D did it in the incorrect order and left steps out. She was shocked to go to a medical spa like mine and have a poor experience. And I was shocked as well. A quick investigation revealed more than a few cracks in her knowledge base. She was inconsistent, often left out critical steps, and was generally considered a ditz by the rest of my staff. Since then I have implemented multiple steps in the hiring process. When I hired D, I didn't even have a working spa. D was the first person I've ever had to fire. It felt like telling someone they have breast cancer. After that experience, I tried to never ever be in the same situation and have to fire someone. I tried really hard.

The Diva

The Diva was an RN who had worked for twelve years at a snazzy, high-end dermatology practice in Seattle. My two most trusted reps vouched for her. One of them told me that she was the only person he let inject himself of anyone in the city. She presented herself as someone who was a star attraction for any practice. She was impeccably dressed and made-up with enormous cheekbones and extra-plumped lips. That is to say, she was the opposite of me in most every way. She was looking for a "medical director" because she had a small space in another neighborhood, just past the distance of her noncompete area required from her previous practice. She had already Googled my spa and knew it was also outside of that five-mile radius.

I wasn't looking to add an injector but could manage that one day each week. I proposed that to make it work, she could open a satellite office and be my employee. I would cover the costs of the entire digital infrastructure, including spa software, website, marketing, and so forth. She would be able to do what she loved best at both places.

The Diva was the first nurse I had ever hired. I dove right in and hired her and talked with a lawyer later. The first rule of hiring employees, consult a lawyer first. There are laws about this stuff. The lawyer told me that I would need to make some changes in the way we operated. RNs cannot work on their own. They cannot see new patients, cannot do "good faith exams," and cannot decide on or devise any treatments. They can only carry out a doctor's orders. We needed an emergency meeting. When I explained what the law says, what I got was a smile and nod. She had operated independently for twelve years under the dermatologists. She had no intention of being "under" a doctor. But she gave lip service to needing to be compliant with the law. We discussed various options to change our process for new patient intake, but she never followed it. The further down the path I got, the more freaked out I became. I lived in fear that any minor complaint might lead to loss of my medical license. Would she lose hers? No. All actions of a nurse under a doctor are the doctor's responsibility.

She smiled and nodded while passively doing nothing to implement change, all the while using my license to practice medicine illegally. We could not work out a proper arrangement. We parted ways almost exactly after two years, which was when her noncompete expired.

It won't be shocking to hear that she is now in the same small office, practicing medicine solo, under someone else's license.

Liar #1

Liar #1 worked for less than a year doing about 50 percent aesthetics and 50 percent medical dermatology. She was an NP from Canada and wanted a job that was 100 percent in aesthetics. I had just parted ways with the Diva, and my business was growing at a strong clip, so I really wanted to hire someone quickly.

(That was one of many mistakes. I have since learned the very grave tenet of business "Hire Slow, Fire Fast."[7] Wanting to hire someone quickly influences you to make so many mistakes in hiring that you might as well go back and read *Business for Dummies*. Thankfully, I have learned from my mistakes, and there have been so many.)

I reached out to L#1 and immediately started ignoring red flags.

L#1 had worked in Canada for fifteen years in a dermatology clinic. She described herself as having fifteen years of injector experience. At the time, I didn't fully understand that no nurses, not even NPs, can perform injections in the entire country of Canada. She was an assistant to dermatologists who did the injecting. I didn't realize there was such a huge gap between our countries in what these nurses are legally allowed to do. Nurses can't work on their own, but they can inject Botox® anywhere in the United States. Not so in Canada. But the way L#1 spoke, she really put herself out as an expert with even more experience than I had. In fact, she had about one year of experience. Lie #1.

Next: she had no qualms about leaving her employer. She did not feel she owed him anything. Are you sure? Do you need to give him some notice so that he can replace you? She said he was a good guy and would understand. Lie #2. If I trained someone for less than a year, and then she took those skills and left me high and dry with no notice, I would mind. I'm sure he minded.

Then there was the negotiation about hours. I told her my philosophy about work. At my spa, we are a team and a family. I ask my staff members each year what their ideal schedule would be. Then I

---

7   Greg McKeown, "Hire slow, fire fast," March 3, 2014, https://hbr.org/2014/03/hire-slow-fire-fast.

give it to them. Then the team covers for one another so that the spa functions smoothly. They can take as many weeks of vacation as they want, as long as the team can cover. Most of my employees choose to work three to four days/week. They tend to take anywhere from four to eight weeks off each year. When you are working your ideal schedule with this much flexibility, it is easy to add a day here or there to cover your teammate, because (1) you have the extra time and you don't feel stressed about your schedule, (2) you will be paid very well for that added day, and (3) next time, they will cover you when you want to be away. It is a win-win for everyone.

I needed either one person full-time or two people part-time. L#1 told me her ideal schedule would be three days/week. Lie #3. So that's what I offered her. On her first day, she shadowed me as I saw patients. Then the red flags went flying. She smirked during a consult where I was explaining all the different body sculpting options. Apparently, she disagreed with me. The only body sculpting device she knew was CoolSculpting®. We were one of the first spas to introduce Emsculpt, a highly effective device with no risk of the complications seen with CoolSculpting®. This was her first exposure to Emsculpt. I asked her if she would be able to learn the physics of the devices and the studies so that she would be able to explain this to patients. She said she had no problems "selling" anything I had to offer. The fact that we educate our patients and that we don't "sell" was not something that she understood. Giant red flag.

Although she had accepted the terms of the offer letter, she came that first day with the letter unsigned. She said that she would not sign the confidentiality agreement because she had accepted a job at a competing med spa as a "medical director" for two days/week. I would have happily hired her to work five days/week, but she asked for part-time. She said she did not want to give up this other position.

When did you accept this position? She said it had happened after she accepted the position with me. So I looked at the website, and she was already on the website as the medical director there. There was absolutely no way she had just taken that job. Lie #4.

Once I saw the lies flying, we parted ways, on day one. It took practically being smothered in red flags before I was able to figure this out. I have since put in place a longer and more thorough process in hiring. But not in time for Liar #2 or #3. *What about Liar #2 and #3? It was pointed out to me that everyone lies to get jobs. So, I'm leaving that here.*

RN#2

RN#2 had worked in a big hospital downtown until a year prior when she had her second child and quit to stay home. Right after the Liars departed, I got an email from RN#2 asking about getting into aesthetics. After meeting for coffee, I invited her to do an official interview.

During that day, RN#2 followed me through every consultation and procedure I did. She asked great questions and was genuinely interested in learning all of the details. She had a mind for science and seemed to get the physics behind the devices. I thought it went well. Because of my experience with the Diva, I knew to set up proper procedures and supervision for RN#2. I thought she might be the perfect fit.

Once she arrived, she complained constantly to other employees but never brought up her grievances with me or the manager. Though she had many issues, the biggest one was the fact that she wanted to skip her training period! Her contract included a ninety-day training period, and by claiming a few days of training over the months before her official start date, she claimed her training period should be waived.

She performed poorly. She had insisted on being paid as a skilled injector, but she never got the hang of it. She lasted only a couple months.

As a result of this experience, I created a "Successful Injector" checklist. And I go over it with each new NP or PA at the ninety-day review, which is announced far ahead of time. And for now, anyway, no RNs. The logistics of legally managing an RN in a medical spa are just not worth the effort. Lastly, though I have successfully trained one NP and one PA, I'm no longer trying to provide my own injector college, hiring only people who are experienced.

What to do/ask before you have a treatment at any medical spa?

- Who is doing the consultation or good faith exam?

- How long have they been performing the service, and how long have they worked at this spa?

- What kind of license do they have?

- Get recommendations from friends and read reviews. If your friends have had a great experience, you likely will too.

- Once you find a doctor (or a PA or NP) whom you truly trust, ask them who they have treat themselves.

If you go to a medical spa (or any aesthetics practice) and you see only an RN or aesthetician and then have a medical service, that's illegal! Always think about your own safety. Don't do it.

If you have a strange or negative experience, *please* speak with the spa manager or the doctor. This is a huge help to us. Any great manager or owner will want to address the situation and make improvements. This also helps us to know if there is a problem. If you do this, and they don't seem to care, don't go back. There are great spas out there; you just haven't found it yet.

KEY TAKEAWAYS

FROM THIS CHAPTER

1. Research Thoroughly: Before choosing an aesthetic expert, do your due diligence. Look for reviews and verify their certifications.

2. Trust Your Instincts: If something feels off during a consultation or you're pressured into a procedure you're unsure about, it's OK to seek a second opinion. It's crucial to feel comfortable and confident in your chosen professional.

3. Stay Informed: Continuously educate yourself about the latest treatments, techniques, and best practices in aesthetics so that you can make informed decisions.

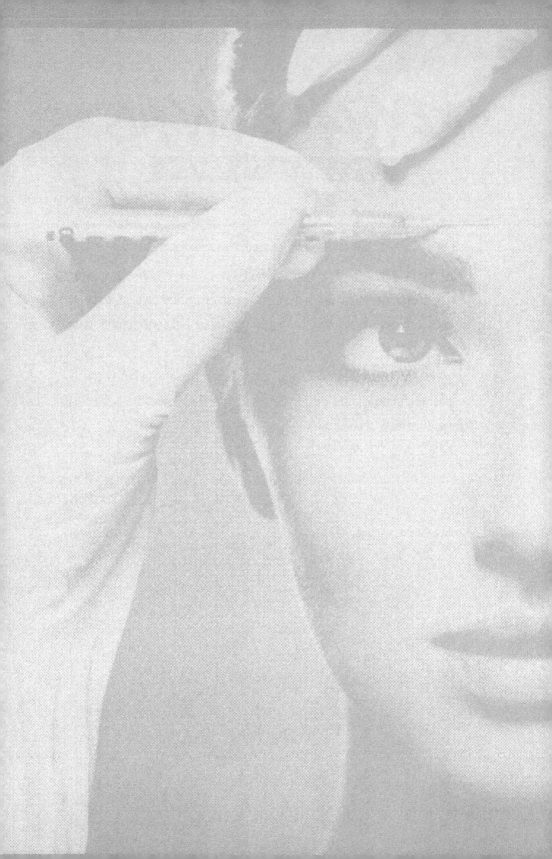

SECTION II

RISKS, FRAUDS, AND PREDATORS OF THE AESTHETIC BUSINESS

This section exposes the dark side of the industry, from fraud to deception.

CHAPTER 4

INDUSTRY CRIMES AND MISDEMEANORS

n our digital era, platforms like Yelp profoundly influence consumer choices. But there's a hidden side to this power. Here I'll uncover the murky interplay between reviews and advertising. Learn how businesses grapple with managing their online reputation amid shadowy tactics. This enlightening read is a cautionary tale, urging discernment in the world of online reviews.

PROTECTION MONEY: THE YELP MAFIA

Many clients seeking aesthetic work depend on Yelp to decide on the best doctor for their procedure. But this is not always going to give you the information you are looking for. Let me tell you about the experiences I've had with this social media. Unlike Google, Yelp has algorithms that control what information and reviews you see on the site.

When I was researching medical spas in my neighborhood, the only place that existed back then had some ugly reviews on Yelp. One woman posted a picture of her battered face, blaming the injector involved and exclaiming, "She did this to me and didn't care at all!" About six months later, that place started advertising on Yelp. Suddenly, they had an almost five-star rating, and those pictures of that bruised-up patient had been taken down. It was a remarkable turnaround. How did such a change in ratings happen?

When I first started in aesthetics and was still in the midst of the harassment at the hospital, I received a scathing personal attack on Yelp. The post profile showed a picture of a famous actor winning an Oscar. The text of the review said some nasty falsehoods about me and my personal life, but in it, the person did not claim to have ever visited my business. There was a picture of the lion lady—a well-known awful picture of a woman with way too much filler in her face—and another picture—a cartoon image of a monkey, slinging feces. The profile itself had just been created, and in it, the person made some statements that made it clear this was Claire. I had no way to prove it, but the details of the post and the profile left no ambiguity. I immediately flagged the review as fake and hit submit.

Then my entire fate was left to the fine people of Yelp. They rarely take down reviews. They have very loose rules, and if *anyone* says your business sucks, it stays. But in this case, because the review did not claim to have ever done business with me, and because of the personal nature of the text, they did take this one down. It was up for six painful days. Yelp does not list a phone number for customer service so that you can contest the review. It won't even let you send in a follow-up message after you've flagged a fake review. You just have to hope someone at Yelp is paying attention.

Soon after this happened, I got a call from Yelp asking me to advertise my business. Now that I had someone on the phone—it was only a salesperson, but I needed answers—I had a *lot* of questions.

What are your policies on fake reviews? Personal attacks? What if this happens again? What should I do? What about my competitor who had bad reviews until she started advertising? The answers were vague but encouraging. "If you advertise with us, we can facilitate your connection with that department." I had no money. I had just started my business, I was in debt, and I really couldn't afford the minimum advertising price they were quoting me. But I also couldn't afford to worry about Claire or any other crazy person out there. I started paying up. That's right. It is protection money.

When you can't fight 'em, what do you do? We ask every patient to write a review. "People love us on Yelp" stickers get sent to us every year. We have a Yelp "Top Med Spa" plaque in our window. I started writing reviews on Yelp for all of my favorite stores and service providers. My kids' orthodontist—five stars! They are awesome by the way. My dentist—five stars! I love her! I know now how important it is to have all the great people who love you *write reviews*! That's the only way to establish your reputation as a great store/spa/professional. If you don't have your lifetime's worth of great reviews to document you're awesome, it is like it didn't happen. Then the one disgruntled person who doesn't like you has all the power. They can ruin you with one terrible review. So, before you read on, take a moment to write a five-star review for your favorite place or person. Right now. I'll wait. They deserve it. You love them. Everyone should know how great they are.

My colleagues who own med spas around the country tell similar stories. Yelp touts their proprietary algorithm. Many reviews are "not recommended" and get relegated to a hidden status. New businesses looking to establish their reputations are dependent on new reviews, but if your patient has never written a review before, that review will be "not recommended." Yelp prioritizes reviews from Yelpers. The more you write, the more the algorithm trusts your review. Even if you're the kind of person who writes ten one-star reviews every day because you hate the world, your review is "recommended." Lovely people who come to a spa for a facial but have only written one five-star review for the ice-cream shop down the street will be "not recommended." Whom do you trust?

Many med spa owners report that the moment they started paying Yelp for advertising, they suddenly had those five-star reviews pop up as recommended. As an advertiser, you get to control what pictures are shown. It is a game changer. Plus your competitors are no longer advertised on *your* page.

Does Yelp advertising generate new business? I don't think so. The actual ads themselves are not widely viewed or helpful. But having great *real* reviews does. No matter how someone hears about you, whether it is from a friend or from a Google search, they will read reviews before making an appointment. Businesses have to play the Yelp game and the review game in general. If paying up for Yelp ensures real reviews stay up on the site, then it will have an impact. What if you're a business that sees clients for the long term and rarely take on a new client? In this case, you likely are not being reviewed very often if at all. But in that case, your one disgruntled person or former employee can make you look really bad online. That's why so many doctors have such bad reputations online. It doesn't reflect reality. But it looks really bad. If you're a doctor, don't Google yourself. If you're not, go ahead and Google your favorite doctor now.

If your favorite doctor has bad or mediocre reviews, go ahead and write something supportive. It's OK; this book can wait. In the middle of writing this chapter, Yelp informed me of a new one-star review. It's pretty bad. A quick glance revealed that this person (who lives in Louisiana?) went to some clinic and had a bad experience with Dr.

Kruger, whoever that is. Hey, this is *not* about my practice! I quickly penned this public response and flagged the review for the fine people of Yelp to take down.

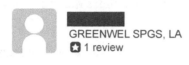

GREENWEL SPGS, LA
⭐ 1 review

⭐☆☆☆☆ 9/30/2019

Worst clinic I have ever seen. The nurse and receptionist are left to do literally everything. The doctor does nothing, and on the rare occasions the doctor comes in to talk it's clear she doesn't want to be there. Dr. Kruger is one of the most impolite I, meanest, self entitled, person with a god complex I've ever met

Comment from Katherine D. of Glow Medispa
Business Owner

9/30/2019 - Hi there. You seem to be referring to a different clinic. There is no Dr. Kruger here. Please consider finding out the correct business to review. Thank you.

After several days with this as the top review on Yelp, there was still no response from Yelp. Was this hurting my business? My overall star rating went down only slightly, because thank goodness, I have a lot of real reviews to balance the overall rating. If anyone reads my response, they will disregard this complaint. When will Yelp respond, if ever? A quick Google search reveals no Dr. Kruger in West Seattle that I can find. As a matter of fact, I can only find one Dr. Kruger spelled this way in all of Seattle—a family doctor who works in an Urgent Care Clinic. Is that where this rotten review should be? That would make more sense! The person who posted says they live in Louisiana—this may or may not be true, as we all move around so much in this economy. Sigh. I must wait for someone or some robot at Yelp to address this. All this sleuthing isn't going to help. And Yelp may just leave it up. As I mentioned, Yelp leaves most of the bad reviews up, even if they are fake. But one of their criteria for taking them down is if you can prove that it is not for your business. I just wait and hope that they figure it out. Meanwhile, that's the top review if anyone looks us up. Fantastic!

Every month or two, I get a call from a sales rep at Yelp. The sales rep has two main jobs. First, to cold-call any and all businesses that appear on Yelp and convince them to advertise. Second is to call every advertiser on Yelp and convince them to increase their monthly spend. Every single business owner I know gets routine visits from these sales reps. They are there to convince you to pay some protection money. When I got my first call, I had already experienced getting beaten up by another gangster, so I was ready to *beg* to be protected. If you agree, you're married to the mob. There's no quitting. You are now scared what will happen if you quit. Will my five-star reviews disappear? Will some other bad guy show up and no one will be there to help?

Many business owners resist signing up as an advertiser on Yelp. They are looking at their marketing budget thinking that it is not a good way to spend those dollars because it won't produce any good leads. Think again. A Yelp budget is not in your advertising/marketing account on QuickBooks. It should be listed under Security with your alarm system and antivirus software. If I were an academic, I would do a study of Yelp ratings analyzed by whether or not the business advertises and how much they pay for Yelp. I'm sure the fine people of Yelp could explain away those findings with lots of allusions to their proprietary algorithms. Let's be real. They are the mafia dons and they know it.

Chapter Postscript: The bad review for Dr. Kruger (whoever he is) was taken down after four days from my account. Thank you to the fine people of Yelp. Thank you very much.

MAFIA WANNABE: REALSELF

Early on in my med spa career, I got advice from the digital marketing company that worked on my website to get myself listed on RealSelf, a website that started here in Seattle primarily for the plastic surgery industry. The idea was to gather stories, information, and before and after pictures from patients who have had cosmetic procedures and give ratings on the procedures themselves and the doctors who perform them. They also wanted to be a source of information for people seeking cosmetic procedures, and they did this by enlisting the very doctors who are getting rated to answer questions from consumers on the site. Doctors are expensive, you might think. How on earth did a tech start-up pay doctors enough money to offer their time and expertise on their site? Would you be shocked to find out that they don't pay a cent?

Doctors don't have a lot of free time. We are usually type A overachievers who overcommit to life by running a medical practice, having families, overexercising, and writing a book on the side. Not that I would know anyone like that. Why on earth would a doctor carve out even more to donate content to a website like this? Well, they learned a few pointers from the fine people at Yelp.

My digital marketing consultants highly recommended I become a "Top Doc" on RealSelf. When I first looked into this, I found that RealSelf did not allow noncore doctors, such as myself, to be listed on the site. Eventually, as the industry was expanding into medical spas, RealSelf realized that it was leaving out a large percentage of the market with that rule. So they expanded to include any physician. The rules on how to become a "Top Doc" and maintain it have changed over the years, but essential to the process is that a doctor answer a lot of questions posed by RealSelf consumers.

At the start, one had to answer all questions. Then they went to a quota each quarter. You also had to have at least five five-star reviews. So by answering these questions, you get a status boost. In a highly competitive field, it helped to be a five-star "Top Doc." RealSelf realized that many of their consumers' questions were going unanswered, so they moved to include nurses as well. This is their free labor source, incentivized by the promise of prestige and a "Top Doc" label.

RealSelf also sells advertising on its site. As a "Top Doc," you will still find your competitors much more prominently displayed on your own page than your own information. If you start paying RealSelf—and their prices are much higher than Yelp—they will delete your competitors. RealSelf promises to supply "highly-vetted, high-quality" patient leads. RealSelf has been at the big plastic surgery and aesthetic conferences taking professional headshots and videos and promising a huge dividend on your ad dollars.

At one of those meetings, they were offering half-off of their usual rate if you sign up for a year. I decided to try it and negotiated it down to six months. If it worked to get the word out about us, I would consider extending. They promised a multitude of leads. I tracked every single inquiry from RealSelf and found exactly one person in six months who came into our spa and had a single service. Meanwhile, I was answering as many questions as I could to maintain my "Top Doc" status. It was like a voluntary hamster wheel.

Eventually, they changed the title to "Top Contributor" instead of "Top Doc." I do have to hand it to them—that's a lot more accurate a term. But it is much less of a motivating moniker. Who needs to be a top contributor of content to a website that is trying to squeeze you like a sponge for both money and knowledge? After six months of this nonsense, we stopped advertising. Luckily, stopping the ads had no negative effects. Unlike Yelp, which knows how to shake you down and leave you in fear, RealSelf has no bite. Most nonsurgical patients are not on the site. It is not a major source of reviews like Google. It just doesn't have the penetration that the others do. It's a wannabe.

RealSelf has plummeted in popularity. The contributors who used to regularly answer users' questions have dropped out. They have failed to become the hub for reviews and information that they were trying for. It is still around, and I am thankful they are not constantly pestering me to advertise anymore.

KEY TAKEAWAYS

FROM THIS CHAPTER

1. Question Transparency: Always be aware that advertising relationships can influence the display or ranking of reviews. Platforms like Yelp should be clear about this, but as readers, we must keep this in mind when evaluating reviews.

2. Beware of Unverified Reviews: Not all reviews are genuine. Some might be fake or written with malicious intent. When reading reviews, look for patterns or signs of authenticity. Remember that platforms should have mechanisms in place to detect and remove suspicious reviews, but many fake reviews remain.

3. Seek Additional Resources: Don't rely solely on one platform for reviews. Business owners are often provided resources to manage their online reputation. As consumers, we should also seek out multiple sources and perspectives before making a judgment or decision based on reviews.

CHAPTER 5

CONSUMER CRIME

T he world of aesthetics is not immune to the dark underbelly of deception and fraud, as evidenced by the tales that unfold in this chapter. As the quest for eternal youth and beauty intensifies, so does the audacity of those willing to exploit the vulnerabilities of medical spas and clinics. From the deceptive tactics of the manipulative Justin to the brazen antics of the so-called Botox® Bandit, we delve deep into the myriad ways unscrupulous individuals seek to gain at the expense of unsuspecting practitioners.

THE MANIPULATOR

Justin (not his real name) came in one day with his husband. They had recently moved into the neighborhood, and he was looking for a new aesthetic provider. He quickly fell in love with our nurse injector and started coming in for treatments. His husband was often with him, sometimes getting treatments himself. Justin had a habit of late cancellations and no-shows. Over time, he accumulated multiple fees, most of which we had waived. But after a pattern emerged, we warned him that we would no longer waive a no-show fee. Soon he repeated the behavior, and we put a no-show fee on his account. His card came back showing insufficient funds. I let him know that he would have to pay the fee and reinstate a valid credit card before returning for another appointment. He told me off in no uncertain terms and said he would never set foot in the spa again.

He stopped coming in, but his husband still came to us for Botox®. I joked with him, "So is Justin OK with you coming in here?" The next day I received a threatening letter from Justin. He complained that I violated the Health Insurance Portability and Accountability Act (HIPAA) by telling his husband that he had been in to the spa on previous occasions. Obviously, the husband had been with him on many of these occasions and already knew this. We did not actually discuss anything about his care. I was trying to acknowledge the tension his visit was causing because his husband had cursed me out and swore he would never do business with my spa again.

I reviewed HIPAA laws with my lawyers. HIPAA is pretty complicated, and we do comply, although technically any medical office that does not take insurance and does not transfer electronic medical records is *not* a covered entity under HIPAA. I felt very comfortable that I had not violated any law.

However, Justin threatened not only a bad Yelp review but also to report me to the state medical board. He wanted a complete refund for all services received by himself and his husband, or he would "put me through hell." My lawyers said that it would be easier to agree to a refund to stop the threats. When the state medical board receives a complaint, they have to go through an exhaustive investigation. I had watched years before when a frivolous complaint had been lodged at one of my colleagues. Though that complaint was completely without merit, it caused a tremendous amount of stress and pain for him—and for me, really, as I felt any of us could be subject to this kind of thing at any time.

Unsurprisingly, all Justin and his husband wanted was the money. Again, I had the same advice from my lawyers. The cost of defending myself against a frivolous claim would be much more than a simple refund.

THEFT AND EXTORTION

You wouldn't think that a medical clinic would need to be concerned with theft and extortion. But, yes, we have to worry about this too. Here's the legal definition of theft and extortion:

> The Revised Code of Washington states that extortion "means knowingly to obtain or attempt to obtain by threat property or services of the owner, and specifically includes sexual favors." *See* RCW 9A.56.110.[8] Under this definition, any attempt—successful or not—to force someone else to give up money, property, or their services, through the threat of violence or some other harm to that person or their reputation, is extortion.

A Google search for Botox® Bandit yielded 279,000 hits. Here are a few examples:

> *Botox® bandit hits Denver medical office* (CO) September 25, 2015

> *Police Seek Woman Accused of Grand Theft after Leaving Botox® Clinic without Paying* (CA) October 12, 2018

---

8   https://apps.leg.wa.gov/rcw/default.aspx?cite=9A.56.110.

Phoenix spa owners seek help from public in catching "Botox® bandits" (AZ) November 15, 2018

"Botox® Bandits" busted: 2 women accused of skipping out on bill at Valley med spa (AZ) February 8, 2019

"Botox® Bandit" Wanted in Washington for Stealing Face Filler

Police say Lauren L. Klavano has received pricey Botox® treatments from spas in Kirkland and Bellevue—but left without paying. (WA) July 25, 2019

"Botox® bandit" arrested, has lengthy criminal history (WA) August 2, 2019

Video shows woman cut hole into glass during med spa heist: police (TX) August 26, 2019

"Soccer Mom" Accused of Breaking into Texas Botox® Clinic with Power Saw to Steal Anti-Aging Products (AZ) August 29, 2019

Botox® Bandit Strikes Again, Pilfering $7,000 Worth of Products (WA) August 30, 2019

Clackamas County woman accused of bolting on Botox® bill. Fifty-eight-year-old Treasa Hansen was arrested for first degree theft. Medical spas say she did not pay for thousands of dollars in cosmetics procedures (OR) October 30, 2019

These stories paint a picture of individuals who seek high-end treatments but disappear without settling their bills. Across the country, headlines from recent years tell tales of thefts and frauds in medical spas. These stories range from those who simply walk out post-treatment without paying to audacious break-ins involving power saws. Such instances not only expose the vulnerabilities of aesthetic clinics but also underline the growing obsession and lengths some individuals are willing to go for antiaging and beautifying treatments. Safeguarding against such incidents is important for practitioners and clinics alike.

THE BOTOX® BANDIT

Let's start with the simple scam, the *Botox® Bandit*. This is happening every day at med spas and aesthetics practices across the country. This is basically the cosmetic version of a dine and dash.

Michelle walked into my spa thirty minutes late for her appointment. She was a teacher and it was Veterans Day, so she was off from work, she said. She said she had Botox® in the past, but it was her first time visiting my business. We took "before" pictures, as we always do. She filled out our medical intake form. We had her contact information. Because Botox® is a pretty quick procedure, we were able to accommodate her despite her late arrival. She had a $420 treatment. At the front desk while checking out, she exclaimed, "Oh, I left my wallet in my car. I'll be right back!" and ran out the door, never to be seen again. The credit card she had on file was declined. The police took a report the next day. They suggested we "send her a bill."

We had her real name, picture, cell phone, and home address. The police knew exactly who she was and where she lived. Nothing was done. The prosecutors did nothing. The last headline above documents the arrest in Oregon of a woman who stole several thousands of dollars' worth of toxin and filler. At least the law is enforced sometimes.

Here's a new kind of combo of online fraud and Botox® banditry that happened to a colleague: A patient got Botox® using three gift cards purchased with a stolen credit card. Then the credit card company charged back the payments, saying it was a fraudulent purchase. Not only did the spa lose the cost of the Botox® and labor, but they had to pay three charge-back fees!

THE CREDIT CARD THIEF

This online gift card fraud happened to us too. A local man had lost his credit card, and his credit card company flagged an online purchase at my spa. The thief used his card to purchase two gift cards online worth $1,000 each. He called us to complain and let us know they were fraudulently purchased. We found the invoice in our system and refunded the money. We also wrote down the gift card code numbers and kept them at the front desk in case anyone ever tried to use them. I thought that this was unlikely, since this would require coming here in person for a treatment. What thief would have the guts to do that? We took the guy's name and number and told him we would let him know if anyone tried to use the codes. He filed a police report.

The next day we received an email from "Guillermo":

Hello team,

I am wondering about BBL, maybe a filler and Botox®.

I am not in a hurry. Please you tell me when you open again and I can schedule an appointment. I already have two gift cards for a total of 2,000.

Thank you for answering,

Guillermo.

Hi there,

Thank you for your inquiry! We are planning to open on March 30th! I do not see any gift cards on your account. Can you provide the gift card numbers or date of purchase so that we can look that up for you?

Thank you,

The Glow Team

Hi,

I attached the gift card codes in this email.

Please let me know if it is everything ok?

Thank you,

Guillermo.

Attached were screenshots of both gift cards, with codes matching the ones we had flagged.

Sorry, those codes are invalid.

Thank you for answering, but Why they are not valid?

Hello team,

I would like to speak with the owner, to try to find a better explanation. I think your answer is a little bit brief and lack of information.

I can go personally too, but I need a better answer to my question.

Thank you,

Guillermo.

We have been informed by the police that these codes have been purchased with a stolen credit card. The credit card company blocked the charge.

Any further threats or communication will be reported to the police.

In our system, it showed that Guillermo had booked three prior appointments but had cancelled all three. He had never been to our spa. He was inquiring about services that few men are interested in, but occasionally, we do have a guy who wants them. Is it possible that Guillermo is a victim here? Maybe someone he knew thought it would be a great gift and gave him $2,000 worth of stolen gift cards? Or maybe he had a friend who knew he wanted our services? If he was innocent, I would have thought he would contact us and apologize for trying to use stolen money and let the police know who gave him the cards. I'll never know for sure, but we haven't heard from him since. I provided this email chain to the victim so that he could give it to the police.

POSTING YELP REVIEWS MALICIOUSLY— OR EXTORTION BY ANOTHER NAME

Carolyn (not her real name) was a new patient who insisted she wanted a particular laser treatment. This is a non-ablative fractional laser that is very versatile and can be used on many different skin types. We sell it in packages of three because you need a series of treatments over several months—it is a great tool to get rid of pigment, smooth the fine lines and wrinkles, and stimulate collagen. We have gotten some great results from this laser, and it has become a mainstay in our arsenal of antiaging tools. But one thing I can tell you is that we never sell this or any other service as a "one and done" treatment. Using safe treatments with low downtime generally means you need several treatments to get to your endpoint.

Carolyn was very excited to try the laser treatment. She said that she would like to do the package but just pay for them "one at a time." She had her first treatment without any difficulty. We did not hear back from her. We send out requests for feedback by text and email to every patient, but there was no response from any of these. Exactly four weeks after her treatment, she posted a one-star review on Yelp, stating that the treatment "scarred her face." I called her immediately and got her voicemail. "Please call me. Please come in for a follow-up. We can take pictures and evaluate what is going on—we will do everything possible to address the issues you are having." I emailed and texted asking her to come in. If there was a reaction like that to this laser, I needed to know about it. Now, many years later, I can tell you we have never had any scarring from this laser.

Carolyn responded to my email stating that she would like her money back, and if I gave her a refund, she would take down her review. She refused to speak with me on the phone or come in for a follow-up visit and pictures. She refused to send us an image showing the "scarring."

This is really the perfect way to get free services! Post a bad review, and offer to take it down only if you get a refund.

KEY TAKEAWAYS

FROM THIS CHAPTER

1. Give Honest Feedback: Give your practitioner a great review if they deserve it!

2. If you have a bad experience, call the office and speak to your provider. They want to help, and they will do anything that can be done to address any issues that come up.

3. It's OK to write a bad review if you have a bad outcome and the office does not respond in any helpful way.

CHAPTER 6

MED SPA MISLEADING
PRACTICES AND DANGERS

I n this chapter, we'll delve deep into the world of medical spas, uncovering the potential pitfalls and unethical practices that can sometimes lurk behind seemingly attractive offers and treatments. From the controversial Bait and Switch tactics employed by some spas to the questionable legality of certain practices, you'll learn how to navigate the aesthetics industry with caution. We'll also expose the dark side of the industry, sharing real-life stories of people who have faced severe consequences as a result of unlicensed or impaired practitioners. By the end of this chapter, you'll be armed with the knowledge and critical questions to ask before undergoing any treatment at a medical spa, ensuring that you make informed decisions for your health and well-being.

BAIT AND SWITCH

One of the medical spas in my area is well known for its Juvéderm® offers on Groupon. I have often wondered how spas like this can stay in business. Injectables are very expensive to purchase. When you see Botox® priced at $8 per unit on Groupon, I can guarantee that the business is losing a lot of money on every person who walks in the door, assuming they are using real Botox®. Eight dollars would not quite cover the cost of buying the Botox®, needles, syringes, and the like, much less the overhead of rent and insurance, and would definitely not pay the doctor or nurse to inject it safely. Groupon itself takes a large portion of the proceeds of each sale. So, how is it possible for the spa to make such an offer? There are a lot of possibilities, and none of them is good.

1. The spa could be purchasing illegal neurotoxin from the gray market. There are many websites selling "Botox®" from Europe or China. Some are simply illegally importing real Botox® from foreign countries. Others are illegally importing Chinese (or other countries') fake Botox®. There are many neurotoxins in other countries that are not FDA approved for use in the United States. Buying them is easy but illegal.

2. The spa could be diluting Botox® or other toxins with extra saline—watering it down. I can't see that they would get away with this for long, as they would have very unhappy customers.

3. They could be using it as a "loss leader." This is when stores purposely offer a product at a loss, in order to upsell customers on more expensive items. They eat the loss, in the hopes that these people will buy other things. Unfortunately,

my research on Groupon customers shows that this probably doesn't happen very often. Spas that are going this way are often throwing a Hail Mary pass before going under.

4. Bait and Switch: This is where the spa uses the coupon to get you in the door, and when you arrive, you find that the original product that you purchased is unavailable, but for more money, you can apply that coupon to something else that has a higher profit margin.

The reps who sell Botox® and Juvéderm® know exactly who buys their product. One day, I asked my Botox® rep about this spa that is always offering a Groupon. I just don't know how they stay in business. I should not have been shocked when my rep said that they haven't ordered Juvéderm® in years. So, how is it that this spa famous for its Juvéderm® Groupon never orders any Juvéderm®?

Juvéderm® is a filler made out of hyaluronic acid, a natural substance that you have in every joint of your body. We like Juvéderm® and other hyaluronic acid fillers because they are recognized as part of you by the body, there are essentially no (or almost no) allergies to it, and most important, they can be dissolved with an enzyme called hyaluronidase if you ever had a complication or an unwanted result.

Some fillers are more permanent. Bellafill is made out of bovine collagen (sourced from calf) with non-resorbable polymethylmeth-acrylate (PMMA) microspheres. It is marketed as lasting five years, but the truth is that it doesn't ever really dissolve. Bellafill is much more expensive than Juvéderm®, but the results are more long-lasting. The downsides are that if you have a complication, such as an arterial occlusion, you can't dissolve it.

WHY RENT WHEN YOU CAN BUY?

When you walk into the Juvéderm® Groupon spa, there is a sign that says, "Why rent when you can buy?" They convert every Juvéderm® Groupon into a down payment on Bellafill. They never have to buy Juvéderm®. The average cost of a syringe of Bellafill is around $1,000 (for a syringe half the size of just about every other filler), and most centers recommend many syringes per treatment, so the total bill when you walk into a spa for Bellafill is often many thousands of dollars, a long way from the cost of a single syringe of Juvéderm®.

Is this legal? Absolutely. Just be warned—if it looks like a deal that is too good to be true, it is.

UNDERSTATING OR OMITTING RISK

Beyond Bait and Switch, there are many pitfalls one faces as a consumer in the aesthetics industry. It is critical to choose your provider carefully and don't believe the hype. Some places will feel like a car dealership—before you know it, you are buying $5,000 worth of fillers you didn't know you needed (and probably don't). Don't be afraid to walk away if you feel pressured into doing something you're not sure about. It is better to walk away and lose a consultation fee than pay for services that you don't want or need—or worse—that make you look ridiculous. If you ask for it, they will sell it to you, whether you need it or not.

We recently had a patient who came for a consultation for dermal fillers. We recommended one to two syringes for the cheeks. This patient then went to another med spa where they recommended five syringes and were ready to inject her that day. They got through the consent process, but the patient couldn't go through with it. She just did not feel comfortable there. When she returned to our clinic for treatment, we went over the entire consent process, including the (thankfully) rare possibility of vascular occlusion. Her eyes widened at this possibility. The other place simply omitted this from the verbal consent. No doubt, they have it in the written form you must sign to have the procedure. But unless you ask, you won't hear about it from them. We have found that very few patients have ever heard of this before—even patients who have had filler many times in the past.

Vascular occlusion is the most feared complication of injectable dermal fillers. Fillers are all forms of a gel. If it were to get into a blood vessel, it could block it. This can lead to tissue necrosis (where a portion of the skin dies from lack of blood flow). This should be a very rare event. This is why we will only use hyaluronic acid fillers at my clinic. Hyaluronic acid fillers are dissolvable with an enzyme called hyaluronidase. We keep a bunch of that in our fridge. As of this writing, we have yet to have caused an occlusion in our clinic. But we have a protocol to follow if—God forbid—this were to happen. We also have an ultrasound device to assist in emergencies. Vascular occlusion and the possibility of it should keep you up at night if you're an injector. If you are getting a consult for fillers from someone who doesn't even mention it, and acts like they're a pro so it can't happen to them, run in the other direction. This can happen to anyone, even if they are ridiculously careful.

This is also why I believe non-dissolvable fillers should be avoided. If you have an occlusion, you're out of luck. Your skin may necrose, and you may be disfigured. It also can't be dissolved if you simply don't like the way it looks. Bellafill used to be called ArteFill, but that name didn't sell well. Bellafill is provided in the United States by very few doctors. Many MDs have come out against its use because of these risks. But there are some very prolific providers who inject a ton of it. They often use a "mapper" who sees the patient before the injector does. This person is there to sell as much product as possible. How can you tell a salesperson versus a medical provider? It can be hard sometimes. Ask what their credentials are, and ask who pays their salary. If they are not working for the doctor in charge, that's a red flag.

IF YOU ASK, THEY WILL FILL

Patricia (not her real name) is a longtime patient of mine. She's in her thirties, and she is her own worst critic. That's pretty common—aren't we all? Patricia is more so than most of us and has a degree of body dysmorphia. She always feels like she needs something. She hates the dimples in her cheeks, so for years we have been filling those in with a half syringe of filler about every six months, and she has been very happy. When she comes in asking for more, I will spend the entire appointment talking her out of it. She is a young mom, stressed in her life and her job. I love talking with her. I tell her she is gorgeous—which she is. She always hugs me and apologizes for taking my time, and I tell her she is always welcome.

One day in early 2020 during the pandemic, when I had cut back my schedule seeing patients, she had trouble getting an appointment with me. I woke up one Saturday morning to this email: "Hi Dr. Dee—I went to Med Spa X and did filler because they could get me in … It was a huge mistake. I wasted so much money and will never see anyone else again. I'm having them dissolve it Monday, but I don't even know *where* they should dissolve it. It looks awful. They used FOUR syringes." Attached were before and after pictures where the befores were beautiful and the afters were ridiculous. Everyone is vulnerable to this sort of tactic—promising you will look even better with more syringes—but people like Patricia are especially so. Many spas will inject what you will pay for. The nurse injectors are often paid on productivity. They make less if you spend less. There is no incentive to talk you out of a procedure. It is extraordinarily shortsighted.

Why? Because the patient will never trust you again. They will tell all their friends: never go to that place. And they will never believe you when you suggest something else that might actually be better for their skin. Several more cases in point follow.

PREPAY FOR SIGHT UNSEEN

A patient inquired about our consultations for dermal filler. We told her that we have a nominal consultation fee that acts as a credit if any service is booked within ninety days. Then she asked if she had to prepay for fillers. We answered no; as a matter of fact, we would not even know what to charge without seeing you first. We have to do an assessment in person and have a discussion about your goals before making recommendations. We can't even guarantee that you'll even need fillers! Some people are better candidates for other treatments. The woman on the phone was floored. She had just had the following experience at a very well-known medical spa franchise:

She asked for a consultation that the spa does virtually by video. Unbeknownst to the patient, the consultation was actually with a salesperson, not a nurse or doctor. This online consultant recommended treatment with two syringes of filler. She was told that to book a filler appointment, she would have to prepay $1,500. This was before she even saw a medical provider. She went ahead with the appointment and the prepayment. When she arrived at the spa for the first time, she did not like the feeling she got there. When she met the nurse, she didn't like her and couldn't trust her. She changed her mind. She was then told that the prepayment was nonrefundable. She was out $1,500, but she told us, "Don't worry, my dad's a lawyer, and he's helping me get my money back."

I mentioned this story at a medical conference to a colleague and was told that this franchise is known for this tactic. The virtual consultations are sales pitches, not medical assessments. They require prepayment for all treatments. I suppose there are a lot of people who don't have dads who are lawyers, because this national franchise is hugely successful.

SORRY—WRONG NUMBER

A friend of mine who is a dermatologist saw a patient who had hugely swollen lips from filler placed at a local medical spa. The doc needed to know what kind of filler was placed to decide whether it could be dissolved. When she called the spa that did the original injections, they refused to send any records or speak to her. When she called the spa back, they wouldn't answer the phone. My friend was left trying to dissolve these overfilled lips without any information about what filler had been injected or how much. Luckily, the filler responded to Hylenex, so at least they had used some kind of hyaluronic acid filler.

Every patient has the right to her or his own medical record. When a spa refuses to send them to you or your doctor, they are violating federal law.

DISFIGURED

Another patient came for a consultation who self-described as "Disfigured" at another spa. She is in her late forties and started to dislike the jowls that had started to form in her lower face. This is a really common complaint. It generally results from laxity of the skin and loss of volume, especially in the cheeks. There are a few options for treating jowls and often use a combination of skin tightening, Sculptra®, and/ or filler. At this other spa, however, they suggested Kybella. Kybella is a bile acid used to dissolve fat. It is FDA-approved to treat the fat pad under the chin (submental fat). In general, the jowls are not caused by focal accumulation of fat in this area. On the contrary, it is the loss of fat pads in your face over time that contributes to the overall droopiness. In general, we are very busy replacing the volume that is lost over time and certainly don't want to dissolve the volume you have left!

This patient did not know any of that. The nurse practitioner at the spa treated her jowls with Kybella. The patient reported that this was excruciatingly painful. It happens that there is a nerve right there, where the jowls form. The first side hurt so much, she was practically jumping off the table. She really didn't want to do the other side but thought she couldn't go around looking lopsided, so she reluctantly finished the procedure despite the pain and had the other side treated. Then she waited. Within a month, she realized the disaster that was emerging on her face. She had two jagged linear divots extending from the corners of her mouth to the sides of her chin. She felt like she looked like an angry witch.

We discussed all the options for a solution. Filler could help, but that is a temporary solution, and would at best get her back to what she looked like when she hated her jowls in the first place. Sculptra® can offer a longer-term solution, but the results from that take months. Ultimately, a combination of skin tightening plus Sculptra® might get her to where she really wanted to be. But, at minimum, a bit of filler would at least replace the volume lost for now.

After just one syringe of filler, she was feeling much more herself. She is contemplating her options for the long term and realizes that the filler will dissolve over time. The longer-lasting options take a lot more time, effort, and expense. She asked me how anyone would have done this to her, and I honestly have no answer. Why do some injectors do things that have no scientific basis? Why would they take risks with people's faces? The only thing I can think of is money. Kybella is very expensive.

Much of what we do in aesthetics is "off-label." But this use of Kybella is so far off-label as it is practically in Antarctica. How do you know that? Again, it can be hard, but asking "Is this off-label?" is a great start. If so, ask how often have they done it before and what have the outcomes been. If they are experimenting with off-label use, you should know about it.

FELONY!

Beyond all of the deceptive and unethical practices in aesthetics, there is the criminal. Here is a headline from 2021 in New Mexico:

Vampire Facial Salon Owner Indicted on 24 Felonies after Two Clients Contract HIV[9]

To be clear: this salon owner did not have any type of license to practice medicine. It was a dangerous and dirty illegal operation.

A filler sales rep I know recently told me that she gets calls frequently from people who cannot legally purchase filler. The most recent one was a dental hygienist who lives in the United States now but moved here from the United Kingdom. She was trying to directly purchase filler that she had bought on her own in the United Kingdom, so she could (illegally, of course) keep injecting here in the States. I can report that the big companies will not sell to people who are not credentialed. However, there is a gray market of direct sales of

---

9   "Vampire facial salon owner indicted on 24 felonies after two clients contract HIV," Toofab, June 7, 2019, https://toofab.com/2019/06/07/criminal-investigation-launched-after-two-people-contract-hiv-from-vampire-facials-made-famous-by-kim-kardashian/.

illegally imported filler from other countries. So, just because someone is injecting, it does not mean they are doing so legally.

IS YOUR INJECTOR IMPAIRED?

As is true of the rest of the economy, the med spa industry has its share of impaired practitioners (providers who suffer from any physical, mental, or substance-abuse problem that interferes with their professional abilities). Because these injectors operate outside of any organization, there is very little oversight as to their abilities to care for others or for themselves. Where do you find out whether your injector is qualified to practice medicine?

Here are some real-life examples:

Injector A is an NP in a state where NPs can practice independently without oversight of a physician. She is a drug addict in recovery. She lost her license years ago and went through rehab. She got clean and got her license back, and that is when she opened her med spa. She has been an aesthetic injector for a long time and is very successful. She is known to pop the occasional Suboxone during the day while at work. (Suboxone is a pill used in a similar way as methadone.) She claims to practice "dermatology" in business networking events. She is a Bellafill injector who often talks her patients into many thousands of dollars of work. Many patients love her, as she is a skilled injector.

Injector B is an MD who is board certified in internal medicine. She herself has a long history of an eating disorder and body dysmorphia. She left her job as an internist to open a medical spa with two friends. She quickly had a falling out with the two founders. Setting up shop on her own, she found three separate beauty spas in which to inject and listed these locations on her own website. However, this also did not last long. None of these beauty spas list her services on their websites any longer. She has since lost her license to practice medicine.

Impairment of medical providers is a very tricky topic. Very few come to light. The only real path to reporting and treatment is through the state medical board (for physicians) or the nursing board (for nurses). But in reality, very few providers are reported. Where med spas are concerned, it is even more unlikely to be reported because the providers are operating independently, with no hospital or other accreditation keeping tabs on them. There is really no surefire way to determine the health of an injector. You can only use reviews and the general pulse of the staff to go on. But even those sources, as I've shown earlier, can be completely unreliable.

QUESTIONS TO ASK BEFORE YOU HAVE ANY TREATMENT AT ANY MEDICAL SPA

1. What license does the provider have? Make sure they have a license to do what they are doing.

2. Is there a doctor in charge?

3. Who is the medical director? Is it a doctor or nurse practitioner?

4. Does the facility use universal precautions (practice sterile technique)?

5. What complications can happen? What happens if there is a complication? What do you do about them? Have you ever had a complication? Is there a doctor present to handle a complication?

6. Is this procedure off-label? If so, how many have you performed, and is it safe?

Be sure to go over the consent form with the provider—and read it! If there is no consent form, run away!

According to the American Medical Spa Association
(presented at a national conference in 2022):
Nearly 15 percent of injections are performed by unlicensed people—
aestheticians, medical assistants, etc.
One-third of these providers don't have a medical director at all.

If you ever have a bad feeling, just leave. Even if you have prepaid! You are not obligated to go through with something you're not comfortable with. The last thing you want is to be a "disaster" headline in your local paper.

KEY TAKEAWAYS

FROM THIS CHAPTER

1. Be cautious of deals that seem too good to be true. Many medical spas offer attractive deals on Groupon, but these can sometimes be a way for them to upsell customers on more expensive treatments or use subpar products. It is important to research the spa and the treatments they offer before purchasing any "deals."

2. Choose Your Provider Carefully: There are many pitfalls in the aesthetics industry, and it is important to choose a provider that you trust and feel comfortable with. Do not be afraid to ask questions, and walk away if you feel pressured into a treatment.

3. Find Out about the Credentials of Your Injector: Make sure that your injector is properly licensed and qualified to perform the treatment. Ask questions about their experience and training, and make sure there is a real medical director or doctor in charge of the facility.

CHAPTER 7

THE PREDATORS

A s a consumer of aesthetic services, you might think that each dermatologist or medical spa offers top-quality services because they have evaluated all of the machines and devices and they have come to offer a certain service because it is the best or works best for their patients in their setting. In this chapter, I will describe the predatory relationship between the big companies and the doctors and spa owners who purchase from them. I hope to convey not only the messy story but also the information that will help you, as a consumer, make the best choices for yourself. If it is hard for a physician to get enough information to make an informed decision, how is it possible for the consumer? I'm hoping this will help.

LASER REPS

The oldest joke in the aesthetics industry is, "How do you get a laser rep to leave you alone? Buy a laser from them." From the day I opened my solo spa, I received cold calls from the laser reps. Laser reps usually work for a laser company, and they are paid primarily with commissions on sales. Most of them are like vultures, hovering over a dead carcass until it is picked clean to the bone. They are not "customer service reps."

The first rep to walk into my tiny little spa was the Soccer Dad rep. Soccer Dad was a guy around my age who lived in my neighborhood. I would later run into him on the local soccer fields when our sons played on opposite teams in club soccer. He saw that I was new to the industry, and I believe he thought he could tell me anything and I would believe him. He was touting a machine that was supposed to tighten skin and kill fat. Plus it had an add-on IPL attached which could treat brown and red spots on the skin. It was the first device I had in my office for a live demo. I had two friends as models, one of whom is an NP. First, we did a treatment on arms. It worked by vacuum suction and radio-frequency (RF) heating, and the handpiece was a bit heavy, and it took a lot of strength to get through one arm. That took almost half an hour, and we still had another arm to go. I remember thinking right off the bat that if I bought this machine, I'd get a workout in every time I did the treatment. What would it be like to do that every day, more than once? If I decided to delegate someday, who would want to do that all day long? My first note to self: don't buy anything you wouldn't be able to tolerate operating yourself.

Meanwhile, I thought, how, exactly, is this going to burn the fat? When you heat the skin up to a certain temperature and keep it there, it can stimulate the fibroblasts in the skin to make collagen, a process that happens over four to six months. Over time, that can tighten skin. But the way this device worked, it could not possibly heat deep enough to get to the fat or long enough to kill fat cells. He was sweaty by the time he was done with the first model and happily declared that she would see a benefit if she got more treatments. I asked for the names of three people who had the machine to call for references. If the reviews were good, perhaps she would go get more treatments at a local spa.

Meanwhile, he got to work using the device for skin tightening in the face. He did half of the face of my NP friend and then held up a mirror, claiming an immediate tightening effect. "That's edema," I replied. The skin is a little swollen. That's not tightening. True tightening takes months to build collagen and elastin. Not minutes of heating. You could get the same effect from a sauna.

In the next few days, I called all three references he provided. The first person I called was a well-known aesthetic doctor and trainer in another state. He told me that he was given the device *gratis* from the company and that he didn't use it. He gave me lots of advice, most prominent of which was "don't buy that machine." The second person I called warned me not to buy that machine and to not do business with Soccer Dad. She told me to call another guy who is an independent rep. She also gave me the lowdown on a few other companies. We'll hear more from her later in this chapter. The third reference was a local spa in Seattle. By this time, I knew I was not buying this machine, so I decided to secret shop the service. I called the spa saying that I had had the service at another place out of state and liked it and was trying to find a place where I could continue. At first, they quoted me an incredibly high price. When I demurred, they immediately cut that price in half. When I thanked them for the info, they did their best to get me to come in for a free consultation. If you ask for references, the expectation is that the person will give you their very best references. If Soccer Dad had no better than this, the device was clearly a dud.

The next rep who visited was selling a microneedling pen called Dermapen. When I mentioned to her that I had demoed the previous device, she said, "If you want one of those, I can get you one real cheap—I know a couple of people who are trying to get rid of theirs." Enough said. This would become a recurring theme—if others in the industry are trying to sell a used device at a cheap price, you have to ask, why? Is it poorly made? Is it because you can't get good results from it and people want their money back? Perhaps that's a sign that it is not such a great deal after all.

The Dermapen pen rep was actually a very nice person and quite informative. Dermapen was going through some rough times back then, and she ended up working for three different companies in a matter of months after I met her. For a while, she worked for a company called Eclipse. They made a competing pen to the Dermapen, and I actually owned one of those, so she became my rep for a nanosecond until she was gone.

Soccer Dad was now working at Eclipse and hired Callie (not her real name). Callie also lives in my neighborhood, and I felt so very lucky to have met her. I was expanding and looking for an aesthetician to work with me, and Callie knew everyone. She spread the word, and pretty soon, I had résumés showing up in my inbox every day without ever having placed an ad. To this day, I am indebted to Callie for helping me to find one of my best and most loyal aestheticians.

One day, however, Callie was trying to get me to switch from the Growth Factor serum I used (which I liked for its high quality and effectiveness and safety) to the one made by Eclipse. She claimed that the Eclipse Growth Factor was human growth factor made from human bone marrow. That this was a medical impossibility did not slow her down. Reps tend to say what their company trains them to say. If they're not listening particularly closely and they promulgate some looser version of those words, they might not even know they are making this stuff up. When I asked for details about how this

Growth Factor was harvested from humans, she ran into a brick wall in her answers. She knew she was caught. The problem is, once I've been lied to, I just can't trust that person ever again.

The first device I ever bought was a microneedling pen. There are many of these devices on the market. Back then, none was FDA approved for skin rejuvenation. Although this procedure had become very popular in a short amount of time, none of the companies had bothered to go through the approval process. I researched and thought I had found a high-quality device called MDPen. This one did not have a local rep and was sold out of a medical device company on the East Coast. The rep who responded to my query was full of information. He was willing to send me the device to demo and would follow up with an in-person training if I purchased the device. If I decided not to purchase, I could return it at no cost. He shipped it to my home. That should have triggered suspicion, but I was naive still. Medical devices can't be shipped to a residential address. They must be purchased by a doctor and shipped to a medical office. After I decided to buy it, he set up an in-person training, where he was to fly to Seattle himself from Atlanta. As the training got closer, he stopped responding to my phone calls and emails. At the appointed time, he was a no-show. In the end, I used the device for less than a year when it self-ignited and literally blew up in smoke. That's when I traded it in for a different pen. By that time, I had learned that these companies mostly made money selling the sterile disposable tips needed for each treatment. Back then, none of the microneedling pens were FDA approved, so the companies were all creating cheap Chinese devices and making money getting you to buy the tips. Now there are several high-quality FDA-approved or FDA-cleared devices on the market. Most places now use high-quality microneedling pens. (For updated recommendations, check the online content at medspamayhem.com.)

Pete (not his real name) walked into my spa one day without an appointment and wanted to speak with me directly, but I was booked with patients. He stayed at my front desk long enough to grab my attention as I walked into a room to see a patient. I told him I was busy. By the time that patient and I had wrapped up, he was still there at my front desk. He immediately launched into his pitch. In one sentence he spoke about a chromophore (pigment in the skin) as the target for a kind of laser that does not have a pigment chromophore. When I pointed out that the chromophore of this laser was water (and not a color), he started arguing with me. When I finally got him to admit his error, he backpedaled and confabulated. And I kicked him out. If you don't know your physics and physiology, these guys can tell you anything, and how would you know they weren't lying? Providers who are not physics or physiology geeks, how would they know he's lying? They don't.

Jake (not his real name) is another rep who worked for at least five companies (that I know of) in only four years. One day he walked into my spa without an appointment. He worked for a company called Merz at the time. He wanted me to buy his version of Botox® and fillers that I had decided not to use. He told me he could give me some free samples to try but would require me to go through a training with him. That's right, he was going to train me to use them. I was part confused and part incensed. I was an MD and make a living injecting actual patients full-time. He is a sales rep with no credentials to inject into a human being, and he was going to train me? "What qualifies you to train anyone to inject fillers?" His answer was a wondrous "I've been trained to train injectors such as yourself." That might have been the biggest lie I've ever heard from a rep. And I kicked him out.

By the way, Jake and Pete (not their real names) are well known in the industry. They all have changed jobs innumerable times since

I opened my spa in 2015. I told them to never call or step foot in my spa ever again. When I tell these stories to other reps and other doctors, they all know exactly whom I'm talking about. My spa is not the only one they've been kicked out of.

One day, in 2018, I could hardly believe my eyes, but there's Jake standing at my front desk again. He introduced himself to me as though he had never been here or met me before. "Nice to meet you, Dr. Dee! I'm your new Prescriber's Choice rep!" Now I was bummed. I work with Prescriber's Choice to provide prescription topicals to my patients. I was stuck with him. For almost a year, all of my orders had to be placed through him. Then, surprisingly, he was fired. I'm not sure where he is now, but these guys move around in the industry just like pedophile priests move around parish to parish. I'm sure he'll surface again.

AND THE COMPANIES THEY WORK FOR

COMPANY C

Every company has a culture, and most laser companies have a sell-at-all-costs culture, regardless of the buyer. Company C has the reputation of being the absolute worst in the industry. At a big laser meeting, I met a doctor from California who was looking for help. She had a general practice and had heard that bringing in aesthetics to a medical practice could help bring in some extra money. She had not been to any aesthetics courses and had no training in lasers when a Company C rep talked her into not just one or two but *seven* lasers at a cost of over $1.5 million. She had no experience and no training, not to mention no idea how to run an aesthetics business, and now she was trying to service this massive debt with no aesthetic patients. She told me that she was taking all her income from her medical practice to make payments on the lasers. She had been unable to reach anyone at Company C to help her market her new services. They would not take any of the machines back, and now she needs to sell them or go bankrupt. The Company C rep will not return her calls.

Company C has among the highest recertification costs in the industry. If you purchase a used laser, "recertification" is a process the company that makes the device requires, in order for them to ever service it or sell you any components or consumables associated with it. Recertification is a set price regardless of whether the device has been used once or thousands of times. This can cost $20–40K depending on the device and the company. The laser companies use proprietary parts and software that will not work without recertification. So, almost all used lasers are eventually useless without recertification. Because of this, it makes used lasers much less attractive to buyers. Once you are in the industry for a while, you realize just how much help you need from the manufacturer. Lasers are not like cars—you can't just go to any mechanic and have them fixed. Laser companies make it very difficult to get service or parts or consumables if you didn't buy the device from them.

Back to our friend in California, she has seven brand-new lasers that she can only sell at fire-sale prices. So, selling them won't get her out of debt. And those of us in the know would never do business with this kind of company, so these lasers are even harder to sell with lower demand.

Another physician told this story when Company C bought out a company that he had been working with for years:

> Never hear much good about Company C, but today they cemented my decision not to ever purchase anything from them! I offer the XYZ procedure, which they recently

bought out. I wasn't hopeful that the change would be good for anyone offering the procedure, and that was confirmed today. Although they've changed absolutely nothing about the kit that you need to purchase and aren't offering anything additional in the way of support or marketing, they raised the price of the kit from $899 to $1,599!! The rep I spoke with today told me that they decided to make the change because they realized some practices were charging a lot for the procedure, so they felt that they should raise the price of the kit. I'd be okay with maybe a $100 price increase, but this seems a bit ridiculous. Glad I don't currently own any of their devices, and this makes clear that I never will.

Company C has become one of the biggest laser companies in the country in part by buying other laser companies. After Company C purchased Company D a decade ago, it gradually changed the way these popular lasers functioned. One tricky sleight of hand had to do with its yearly service contract. Lasers are very sensitive machines. They can be damaged very easily and can be very expensive to repair. Yearly service contracts for devices range from $8K to $15K/year. Most of us would prefer not to pay that yearly cost, but it is a disaster if your laser breaks down, and not only does it cost more than that to fix, but you don't have a loaner to use while yours is being fixed. So, most of us pay up. Company C makes it essentially mandatory. They started using a software key that they distribute each year in a USB drive that must be plugged into the machine. If your USB is expired, your machine won't work, even if there is nothing wrong with it. Imagine purchasing a high-performance race car for $150K, and they tell you that the key won't work in one year unless you pay an annual service fee of $15K. That's how Company C operates.

Company C itself was purchased a few years ago by Company E, a company best known for its high-quality imaging machines. Since I had worked with Company E for many years in radiology and knew it as a company with very high standards, I wondered whether it would change the culture at Company C. Company E announced after two years that it was selling C to a private equity firm for a total purchase price of $205 million in cash. Only two years before they paid $1.6 billion for it. Now owned by private equity, Company C continues to have the same stellar reputation it had before the acquisition.

COMPANY M

I have met with a few Company M reps in the past but never seriously considered an actual purchase, though they do make some quality devices. Company M and Company C tend to vie for most despicable in the rep department. Someone in one of the sales meetings for Company M captured this slide on their phone. The poor spelling and grammar alone would merely annoy me. But the rest—I'll just leave this here for you to judge.

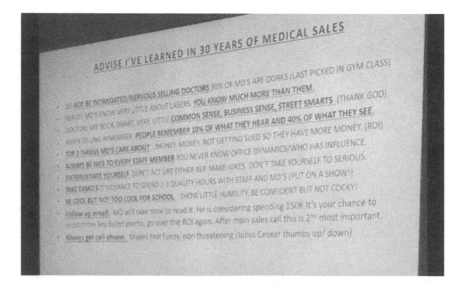

Can't read that? Well, we've made it easier—poor spelling and all:

ADVISE I'VE LEARNED IN 30 YEARS OF MEDICAL SALES

- DO **NOT BE INTIMIDATED/NERVOUS SELLING DOCOTRS** 90% OF MD'S ARE DORKS (LAST PICKED IN GYM CLASS)

- REALIZE MD'S KNOW VERY LITTLE ABOUT LASERS. **YOU KNOW MUCH MORE THAN THEM**.

- DOCTORS ARE BOOK SMART, VERY LITTLE **COMMON SENSE, BUSINESS SENSE, STREET SMARTS** (THANK GOD)

- WHEN SELLING REMEMBER: **PEOPLE REMEMBER 10% OF WHAT THEY HEAR AND 40% OF WHAT THEY SEE**.

- **TOP 3 THINGS MD'S CARE ABOUT** ... MONEY, MONEY, NOT GETTING SUED SO THEY HAVE MORE MONEY. (ROI)

- **ALWAYS BE NICE TO EVERY STAFF MEMBER** YOU NEVER KNOW OFFICE DYNAMICS/HOW HAS INFLUENCE.

- **DIFFERENTIATE YOURSELF** DON'T ACT LIKE OTHER REP. MAKE JOKES, DONT' TAKE YOURSELF TO SERIOUS.

- **TAKE DEMO'S** IT'S CHANCE TO SPEND 2-3 QUALITY HOURS IWTH STAFF AND MD'S (PUT ON A SHOW!)

- **BE COOL BUT NOT TOO COOL FOR SCHOOL** SHOW LITTLE HUMILITY. BE CONFIDENT BUT NOT COCKY!

- **Follow up email**: MD will take time to read it. He is considering spending 150K it's your chance to re-pitch the key bullet points, go over the ROI again. After main sales call this is 2nd most important.

- **Always get cell phone**. Makes text funny, non threatening (Julius Cesar thumbs up/down)

Company M has denied it was them and tried to suppress this from making the rounds. But this little gem of a slide made its way to most every MD in aesthetics. I may be a dork, but I grew up in

New York City in the '80s. I'll put my street smarts up against the best in the biz, bucko. I was informed by my editors that the rest of my color commentary about this slide was perhaps a little spicy for this manuscript. So, you can read the slide and feel free to imagine a line-by-line slam response.

FAKE CONSUMABLES

A consumable is literally a product or part that is used up in a procedure. For instance, the syringe and needle, gauze, and alcohol that are used to inject Botox® are all consumables. And the Botox® itself is a consumable. For years, there were essentially no consumables with lasers. Lasers are devices that emit a narrow beam of single-wavelength light. They were expensive to purchase and maintain, but there were no parts that were used up during a treatment. Eventually, the laser companies created laser tips that need to be changed out at various intervals or every time. Since these tips can touch the patient or act as guides for the treatment, it makes sense that they would wear out over time.

Then the RF devices surged in popularity. These machines are much cheaper to manufacture. Many of them require a grounding pad to be placed on the patient. That too is a consumable. RF microneedling devices require a sterile needle tip to be used for each treatment. These are needles that can become dull, but most importantly, are contaminated with a person's blood. Those can be up to $150/tip. This is what I call a real consumable. Something that simply must be discarded and cannot be reused.

CoolSculpting® is famous for creating what I call a *fake consumable*. This is something that the manufacturer requires to be replaced, even if there is nothing wrong with it or it is not "used up."

CoolSculpting® charges hundreds of dollars for new applicators each treatment, when the device could easily be designed without this. The thing that is maddening is to look at a piece of clear plastic and know that you are being charged hundreds of dollars for something that costs a tiny fraction of that to manufacture.

The most egregious practice skips the fake consumable and goes straight for a per-use fee. Company S is notorious for this. For their lasers, they charge a per-use fee. They issue credit cards that must be installed on the machine, or they will cease to function. Each card carries with it so many uses. One card allows forty minutes of use per patient. If the patient has to use the bathroom in the middle of a session, you lose that time, as it cannot be paused mid-session. If there is an emergency and you have to stop, you're out of luck. Similarly, if you have a short treatment, you can't save your minutes for the next person.

COOLSCULPTING®

Probably one of the most famous aesthetic procedures is CoolSculpting®. This was the very first fat-destroying device that actually worked. CoolSculpting® works by freezing fat. It was developed by a Harvard dermatologist who founded a private company called Zeltiq in 2005. Zeltiq was quickly successful using a direct-to-consumer model in which they charged a very high (fake) consumable price and directed much of that money to direct marketing.

Early adopters to this model were very happy and did very well with the device. There was nothing else like it—and it really could kill fat. Over time, Zeltiq sold more and more of these devices, flooding the market. Each device could only freeze one applicator full of fat each treatment, and a patient might need four or even six applicators full to completely treat an area. So the company encouraged each provider to purchase more machines (calling it "dual sculpting" if they had two, etc.). Some offices would buy four or eight or even more CoolSculpting® devices, so they could shorten the total treatment time for patients and make more money per hour, as long as the machines were busy. And this increased revenues for Zeltiq because they charged so much per applicator.

As CoolSculpting® became better known and more people Googled it, Zeltiq started pitting its doctors against one another in competition, as a prompt to sell more devices. On its provider finder, the more machines you bought, the higher up you would appear on the search list. Over time, they also dramatically increased their applicator prices.

Back in 2015, providers were already becoming disgruntled by the way they were being treated. One of my original connections who told me not to buy that original device told me also *not* to buy CoolSculpting®. She said it was getting harder and harder to make a go of it.

Meanwhile, millions of people were getting their fat frozen and having issues. The biggest one was uneven, wavy results. One of the problems with the technology is that you can only kill the fat that you can suck into the cup. The adjacent fat is left untreated. So if you run out of money, or if the adjacent fat is simply outside the treatment area, you'll have a noticeable difference between the treated area and the adjacent fat, often resulting in "shelfing" with a divot where the fat was treated and full fat next door. We treated several of these cases early on with our devices, but the wavy, lumpy results are tough. Some bodies are better candidates for this treatment than others—it really depends on the distribution of fat. Providers who are really good at patient selection have much better outcomes.

The worst complication of freezing fat is paradoxical hyperplasia of the fat (paradoxical adipose hyperplasia or PAH). The fat in this case grows instead of shrinks. And with PAH, the new fat is rock hard and does not easily respond to traditional treatments (like liposuction) and often must be surgically excised.

COOLSCULPTING® IN THE NEWS

CoolSculpting® had some major setbacks in 2021. First there was the much-reported lawsuit by supermodel Linda Evangelista, who claimed that CoolSculpting® left her disfigured:

New York Times: Supermodel Linda Evangelista
Says Cosmetic Procedure Left Her "Disfigured"[10]

The model had CoolSculpting® treatments to multiple areas of her body. There are a few published pictures, but she claimed that she had PAH and was left disfigured by the procedure. It is unclear whether she had PAH in multiple places or whether she had them surgically removed. I've often repeated in my aesthetics career that "nothing in aesthetics is worth risking any permanent harm." Well, this would be why. There is also at least one class-action lawsuit claiming the same issue that the supermodel is claiming:

CoolSculpting® Weight Loss Procedure Customers File
Class Action Lawsuit Alleging Bodily Deformation[11]

The maker of CoolSculpting® settled their case with Linda Evangelista in 2022 for $50 million. As part of the deal, they did not have to

---

10   Christine Hauser, "Supermodel Linda Evangelista says cosmetic procedure left her 'disfigured,'" *The New York Times*, September 23, 2021, https://www.nytimes.com/2021/09/23/us/linda-evangelista-lawsuit-paradoxical-adipose-hyperplasia.html.

11   Jessy Edwards, "CoolSculpting® weight loss procedure customers file class action lawsuit alleging bodily deformation," topclassactions.com, June 1, 2021, https://topcl-assactions.com/lawsuit-settlements/medical-problems/coolsculpting-weight-loss-customers-class-action-lawsuit-abbvie-bodily-deformation/.

admit any wrongdoing. Meanwhile, the *New York Times* published an article on April 16, 2023, about how the rate of PAH is actually much higher than Allergan claims:

A Beauty Treatment Promised to Zap Fat.
For Some, It Brought Disfigurement[12]

Then a week later on April 22, 2023, the *Times* published their investigation of how often PAH occurs. They contend it could be as much as 50 percent.

Just How Rare Is a "Rare" Side Effect of
a Fat-Zapping Procedure?[13]

The second controversy regarding CoolSculpting® is very different. The device companies are always innovating and improving their devices. When they make major improvements, they will often issue a new device or upgrade and convince current clients who own the first device to "upgrade" to the newer device. I have several devices that are the new and improved versions of a device I owned previously. You have to know when to bite the bullet and spend the money for the upgrade and when to sit tight with a device that already works for you. This can be tough, and if you really love a device, you are likely going to want to buy the upgrade.

---

12   Anna Kodé, "A beauty treatment promised to Zap Fat. For some, it brought disfigurement," *The New York Times*, April 16, 2023, https://www.nytimes.com/2023/04/16/style/coolsculpting-side-effect-risks.html.

13   Anna Kodé, "Just how rare is a 'rare' side effect of a fat-zapping procedure?," *The New York Times*, April 22, 2023, https://www.nytimes.com/2023/04/22/insider/coolsculpting-investigation.html.

Class 2 Device Recall—CoolSculpting® Elite System[14]

An "upgrade" to CoolSculpting® was introduced, called CoolSculpting Elite. Existing CoolSculpting® providers were pressured to buy the upgrade but provided no studies showing that it gave any improved outcomes. Many followed suit and bought the new device, trading in their old devices. Soon after, there was a problem with the FDA (because of side effects and a few burns), and the new machines were halted. For months, these people couldn't get their money or their old machines back. Suddenly, these CoolSculpting® providers could no longer provide any services and had no revenue. Recipe for mutiny.

In a lot of ways, buying a body contouring device is like betting on a horse race. You have to do a lot of research, but in the end, it is still a very expensive gamble. As of today, the two most effective body sculpting devices are CoolSculpting® and Emsculpt Neo. Obviously, I have been betting on Emsculpt for a long time. Because of its safety profile and efficacy, I'm sticking to that until something proves to have even better outcomes. For the latest recommendations on body contouring, check out our online content at medspamayhem.com.

PREDATORY LENDERS

Equipment financing can be stressful. Many people know how hard it is to spend your life savings as a down payment on a house. Imagine spending $250K for a laser. It takes your breath away. The equipment companies that want to take your money are often allied with an equipment financing company. They are not banks but sometimes call themselves banks. They are there to make you feel like you're getting

---

14   "Class 2 device recall CoolSculpting elite system," accessdata.fda.gov, 2021, https://www.accessdata.fda.gov/scripts/cdrh/cfdocs/cfRES/res.cfm?id=188569.

a great deal, but if this were a mortgage, they would be shut down for their predatory lending practices. But mortgage laws do not apply.

These lenders offer a higher interest rate than any commercial bank, and they embed huge penalties for prepayment. Usually, you will pay *all* the interest due on the entire lifetime of a loan, even if you pay it off early. I met one med spa owner who paid $250K for a device and she is losing money every day trying to make the payments but not doing very much business. She could sell the brand-new device, but few would pay what she paid because they would have to pay a huge recertification fee to the device company in order to use it. If she sells it for a low price, she will still have to pay $40K in interest that would have been due over five years. So she owed $290K from day one of owning a $250K device. That's a 16 percent markup. She could probably sell her device for about $140K, at a $150K loss. And she would have to come up with the cash. So, for now, she keeps going, hoping to make the best of it. The device is actually a good one, so if she figures out a way to market her services, she will probably make it through the next five years.

The collaboration of the laser companies and the predatory lenders is particularly problematic. The laser reps insist their laser is a must-have, and when they've convinced you to buy it, they have in their pocket an automatic loan that makes the sale easy and immediate. Otherwise, the buyer would have to shop around for an equipment loan from a commercial bank. If they did that, they would find out that commercial banks offer exactly this kind of loan and a more reasonable interest rate and more fair terms. Over the years, I took out three different equipment loans at low rates and paid them all off early with no penalty. I am grateful to the rep whom I found early on in my journey because he warned me not to use the equipment financing that the company used. He connected me with a commercial lender.

Why was he helping me? He was an independent rep—he did not work for the company. He just sold the devices. He didn't have any financial stake in his customers taking on the bad financing deal.

How do these predators affect the consumer? Because they've pinned many doctors and med spa owners into a very rough spot, owing massive amounts of money on a bunch of devices that may or may not work. These owners have every incentive to sell you their services whether they work or not. They have loans to pay!

KEY TAKEAWAYS
FROM THIS CHAPTER

Med spas are businesses, with bills to pay. Many of them may have financial incentives to sell you something that may not be in your best interest. Many have fallen into the traps set by these predators. It is important to ask the right questions.

Questions to ask before having a treatment with a laser or aesthetic device:

- What device is it, and what company makes it?
- How long have you used it, and how many patients have you done?
- Can you show me before and after pictures of your own patients?
- Are there any studies showing efficacy?

Then read reviews of that device, not just a review of the spa.

SECTION III

A PERSONAL AND BUSINESS PERSPECTIVE

CHAPTER 8

REFLECTIONS ON LIFE AND BUSINESS

I n this chapter, I talk about working as a physician in breast cancer and my transition to aesthetics. In sharing these stories, I hope to convey the profound impact my patients and I had on each other and the complex emotions involved in both delivering and receiving a cancer diagnosis. I share my stumble into business and a bit about why I feel that I'm still helping people in a profound way through my work in aesthetics.

I REALLY HATE BREAST CANCER

When I worked at the breast center, I read lots of mammograms, ultrasounds, and MRIs. Diagnostic cases included mammograms and often ultrasounds for the evaluation of breast problems. If they were abnormal, I'd speak with the patient and explain the findings and talk about next steps.

"This is a thirty-six-year-old who felt lumps when she was pregnant and then breastfeeding. She recently stopped lactating, but the lumps didn't go away so her OB sent her in." Jennie was my best tech and always succinct with the history. The mammogram showed an obvious, very large cancer. The ultrasound showed the same thing. I took a deep breath.

I walked into the room to find her holding an adorable one-year-old son. "Hi, Dr. Dee," her husband said as he reached out to shake my hand. Rich worked at the hospital, and I had worked with him. He and his wife, Michelle, thought I was about to tell them she had an infection or "clogged ducts" as had been suggested by her OB/GYN. My job was to get them through the next few minutes and days as best I could, without freaking them out but with accurate information. I broke the news as gently as I could without whitewashing and added her on to my schedule that very moment for a biopsy. She was gone before her son turned two.

Sandra was a striking forty-eight-year-old African American woman who had been suffering from depression for the last year. As I explained the findings on her imaging, she looked straight ahead with no expression. She didn't want to know and probably wouldn't have a biopsy. I talked about the size (medium) and how the nodes looked normal (a good sign) and how most women survive and do great when cancers are like that (and they do). She was reluctant but went ahead with the biopsy. When the results came in, I personally set her up with my favorite breast surgeon, who I thought she would respond to. She did, all through the MRI and plans for oncology, right up until the time for surgery when she showed up for her pre-op wire procedure in my office and had a change of heart at the last minute. She couldn't go through with it. "I'd rather die of breast cancer than have my body cut up." I said, "I'm not going to assault you today. You will never have to do anything you don't want to do." I told her that my part of today would be quick and painless—which by this time she knew I would be gentle and truthful. And I somehow cajoled her into going through with the plan. Her lumpectomy went smoothly.

Six months later, I was in the reading room when Sandra popped in. I had just read her first post-op mammogram, and it looked great. She had a big smile on her face, walked straight up to me, and gave me the biggest hug I've ever received. "I cannot thank you enough, Dr. Dee. I have had the most amazing six months of my life. It is like the depression was cut out of me along with the cancer. I thought I was alone in this, but so many friends have been there for me. I had no idea so many people loved me. I'm back in my martial arts class and exercising. I haven't felt this great in years!" I was in tears by the time she finished telling me about her life now. To this day, I don't know whether the otherwise silent cancer could have been contributing to her mental state or whether the outpouring of friendship and love around the diagnosis cured her.

Marian was a nurse at a local hospital. She hadn't had a mammogram in three years because she was the kind of person who took care of others and often neglected herself. She was a nurse and a grandmother, and she just hadn't had time. But she felt a lump and knew she needed to come in. The cancer was pretty big, but worse, she had very large abnormal lymph nodes in her armpit. She would need the works—surgery, radiation, chemotherapy. But her cancer also had some good signs—hormone receptors (meaning it could be suppressed with hormone blockers—a good thing) and negative for some more bad markers, meaning it would be easier to treat than some others. She had a lot of regret in the beginning, about not getting her screening mammograms, about not feeling this big lump sooner. Maybe if she had done all that, we would have found it a lot sooner? We spent a lot of time talking about life and how you can't look back and second-guess now—you can only look forward and be strong. She lost her hair for a while, but the chemo did its job. For every follow-up, she made sure to come on a day I was working, and she visited me every time. One day, I met another nurse at the same hospital with a similar cancer. I was pretty sure they knew each other at work. Because of HIPAA, I couldn't just introduce them, but I asked each of them permission and gave them contact information so that they could connect if they wanted. They were both going through similar issues at the same time, and they were able to share a unique friendship and support each other rather than feeling alone at work. After three years, her visit was brief and happy. She said she was going to go back to screening mammograms but wanted to visit with me anyway and if that would be OK. Of course, I would love to see her any time.

Fast-forward two more years. I had just separated after a fourteen-year relationship. We had three small kids. This was my first day back in the breast center, and Marian was my last patient of the day. She looked amazing despite walking with a cane. After I told her that her mammogram looked great, I asked her how she was doing and what was going on with that cane. She updated me on her life, how she was happily enjoying her grandchildren, and dealing with arthritis in her knee. Then she looked at me and said, "Enough about me, tell me how *you* are doing?" I just broke out in tears and blathered on about my divorce, the kids, how hard it was being back at work. She spent half an hour telling me about her own divorce and life stories and giving me the encouragement I needed to get through that day and the next. At the end, she gave me a huge hug and said, "What a pleasure it is to take care of *you* for a change." To this day, I think how incredibly lucky I have been to know her. By the way, Marian is a true survivor and an inspiration. She's still out there taking care of people, and though we haven't spoken in many years, I am forever grateful for her insight and love.

THE GIFT OF LAUGHTER

My family loves it when I devolve into a fit of laughter and can't recover. I'm too serious most of the time, but when this happens, the whole fam follows suit as they watch me spurt water (or wine) out my nostrils, unable to breathe or swallow.

But that's not the laughter I'm talking about. I'm talking about the men laughing at me around the boardroom. It was really a basement hospital conference room with uncomfortable chairs and no cellular reception where our meetings were held each month, but boardroom sounds better. It was at a board meeting for my radiology group where they laughed at me when I proposed to start a small aesthetic practice within my old practice. It would have cost them nothing, but they laughed me off. It was the day before my birthday, too. The first thing I did the next day was place a deposit on a small room to sublet in a medical suite in West Seattle, my neighborhood, and five minutes from my home. The second thing I did that day was secure my own business and malpractice insurance. The third thing—a domain search. Glowspaseattle.com was available. It was a little long, but it was cheap and I bought it. Before I knew it, I was designing my own website on Wix.com.

If they had said yes, they would own my business now. Except. That group did not flourish after I left. There had been some rough negotiations with the hospital, and, eventually, they all got kicked out of the hospital three years later. I didn't hear about the details until much later. If I had stayed, my business probably would have been sucked into the dissolution of the practice. I'm not sure who had the last laugh, but I definitely received the last buyout.

STILL CHANGING LIVES

People sometimes still ask whether I miss Big Medicine or working in the breast center. It was incredibly rewarding, and I did love my job for a long time. But do I miss breast cancer? No. In aesthetics, I still get to connect with my patients, and I still have some profound effects on their lives. I might not be saving lives anymore, but I know I'm making an impact.

NO SWEAT

Not only do neurotoxins treat wrinkles, but they also shut off the sweat glands. It is normal to sweat when the body needs cooling. But some people suffer from hyperhidrosis, which is a medical condition where the body sweats profusely even when it does not need cooling. Often the sweat is on the hands, feet, underarms, and head, while the rest of the body stays dry. About 2.8 percent of adults in the United States suffer from hyperhidrosis, men as much as women. Of those, about half have axillary hyperhidrosis or severe sweating in the underarm areas. This can be a devastating problem when you are trying to present as professional and calm or romantic and sexy—and there are giant sweat marks in your underarms.

Before toxins came along, treatments for hyperhidrosis were drastic, expensive, painful, and often not all that effective. Toxin treatment is simple and very effective and lasts usually much longer than the typical three to four months we see for wrinkle treatment— usually between six and twelve months. Injections in the underarm are surprisingly painless. The effects usually set in within a few days but may take up to two weeks to have maximum benefit.

One day Avery came in for the very first time asking about treating her sweaty palms. She was in her mid-thirties, had researched it, and was ready to give it a try after many years of feeling embarrassed to ever shake hands. It takes a full vial of toxin to treat both hands, so it is pretty expensive, but it also tends to last a long time—eight to twelve months for most people. I gave her an ice pack to hold in each hand and treated both palms and all of the fingers. It hurts but, thankfully, is a quick procedure. She left, and I didn't hear back from her until almost a year later. I was excited to see her and wondered how it worked for her. She was ebullient. She said that the sweating had completely stopped, and she actually forgot she had even had a problem. Three months after her treatment, she got a big promotion in her job that required a lot of travel and recruiting—a job she would have turned down in the past because of the sweaty palms. She took the job offer, which came with a big raise, and has loved it. She said two weeks ago, she started to feel sweaty in her palms, and she actually thought to herself that she must be getting sick. "I forgot it was a thing." After another week went by and the sweating came back to its full-blown deluge, she remembered. And she booked another appointment. "I never would have taken this job if it hadn't been for the toxin! So the moment I realized the sweating was back, I booked this time to see you again."

EVADING THE STALKER

One day when I first started the med spa, Maria came in for a consult. She was tired and thin and very run-down. She wanted to look better and basically said she would do whatever I recommended because she just wanted to look different. And better. She was going through a divorce, she said. At first, we did some simple injectables, some neurotoxin and fillers, and that had an immediate effect. She loved it. Soon after, she signed up for a series of skin tightening treatments. Every time she paid in cash. Over the months, she revealed the source of her stress. Her soon-to-be ex was stalking her. He was threatening physical harm, and she had fled, and she did not want him to find her.

In that first year, she blossomed like a flower. She gained strength physically and mentally. She looked amazing. Eventually, she offered to pay with a credit card. I asked her, "Are you sure? Is it safe?" "Oh, yes, I took care of him!" I never found out the specifics of that, but I know that the aesthetic treatments were a huge part of her gaining her independence and her life back. To this day, hers are some of the best before and after photos I have ever taken.

HEADING BACK TO WORK

Ellie was in her early fifties, recently divorced and trying to get back into the workforce after a long absence to raise her children. She was anxious and pretty down about the situation. She was competing against much younger people for the same positions and felt the ageism that permeates our society. She also didn't have a ton of money to spend.

We talked about what would give her the most bang for her buck to get her back into the workforce quickly. We decided together that some toxin for the 11's and wrinkles around her eyes would be number one. We then tried just a bit of filler for her cheeks. The difference was remarkable, and I think she left the spa feeling like it was worth it. The next time I saw Maria, she had landed a great job. She had bought new clothes. From that time on, she was always one of the most put-together patients I've ever had. Her confidence and style are matched by her smile and her kind personality, and she has succeeded in competing with others decades younger. Feeling confident in your appearance does wonders for your overall confidence and success in life.

ROMY AND MICHELE

When my kids were younger, I took them to see a live performance of *Romy and Michele's High School Reunion, The Musical.* Don't judge me—it was fantastic! If you don't know which one of them invented Post-its, please go rent the movie. It is totally worth it.

In the musical version, the finale (*spoiler alert!*) is a superb heart-warmer. Our protagonists have finally figured out their passion, and we see them using their flair for fashion design turned into a full-blown store. We see various characters wander into the store for fashion help. My favorite is a middle-aged mom who needs an outfit for her daughter's wedding—that her ex is coming to with his new girlfriend who is her daughter's age. We see her go in the back and come out wearing the perfect outfit that is gorgeous and sexy and she is all smiles. The number is called "Changing Lives One Outfit at a Time."

My daughter sitting next to me whispered in my ear, "Mommy—that's what you do!" I had never thought about it that way, but I have ever since. See the show if you can. It is hilarious.

BLACK-AND-WHITE COOKIE HEAD

SMALL BUSINESS FOR DUMMIES

I was looking to hire a manager for the spa for the first time. I created a job description and placed an ad. Since I had never had a manager before, and I didn't have huge revenues, I didn't have a very high-paying job to offer. As a result, I had a lot of résumés for people with no experience. Most of them had worked in sales/retail. Few had any experience in anything medical or managing people. I sorted through about eighty résumés and narrowed it down to about four.

The first woman I interviewed sounded great on the phone. She was engaging and articulate and had worked in retail. She had bonus points for living in our neighborhood and was within walking distance of the spa. I met her in the morning before we opened. As I spoke with her, my staff members who were working that day filed in to get ready for the day. As they arrived, I introduced them to the candidate. We had a decent discussion, though I came from the meeting feeling ambivalent.

One of my aestheticians was in the staff room after she left, and I asked her what she thought. She made an exaggerated face with her eyebrows arching way up into her forehead and said, "Wow." The candidate had very thick drawn-in eyebrows that arched halfway up her head, like a clown. It was distracting for me and made me feel old, but I had been willing to ignore it. She also had nails that were at least an inch longer than her fingers. When I asked her how she typed on a keyboard, she said she "gets by." My staff all felt that these things were incredibly distracting and that this did not represent our business, which is, of course, all about aesthetics.

This gets into a very difficult area. I would never discriminate on the basis of race, sex, and sexual orientation. But eyebrows and nails? I had to look that up—is that legal? Well, actually, from what I could tell—yes—as long as the appearance isn't due to a deeply held religious belief. She wasn't in the running anyway because of her résumé. Finding the right person is so very hard.

The next candidate was a manager at Sephora who had a little more experience but, again, nothing having to do with medicine or science. When she arrived, she had the left side of her head dyed black and the right side dyed stark white, with a part down the middle. I was immediately reminded of the black-and-white cookies in New York when I was a kid.

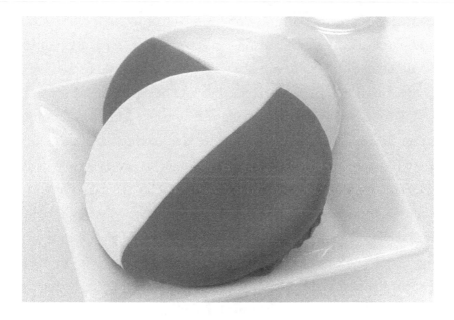

I can hardly remember the conversation. I don't even eat cookies, but I found myself nostalgic for those big NYC black-and-white cookies. Have you not had one? When I picked up my kids from school, I described it, and they all said practically in unison, "You mean, like Sia?" Huh. It was clearly a thing, and it had passed me by. Although by the time this interview was taking place, Sia had moved on from that hairdo. I really felt like an old lady.

What was I saying? Oh, right. I really don't remember the conversation. Just the hair. Eventually, I ran through all the résumés with no viable options. Then one of my employees handed me a résumé from someone who had stopped by the spa. She lived in the neighborhood and had been in once or twice for services. My employee said, "She's a keeper!" She was described to me as someone who was really enthusiastic about getting into the aesthetics industry. Smart and capable, she would be worth speaking to.

Penny (not her real name) was warm and had a great smile. She was from California and had a valley-girl persona, but she was really excited about the opportunity. She was willing to learn the industry and start from the ground up. She was far and away the best candidate I had found for the position. She was young and would be managing people twice her age. But I decided to give her the job.

Penny started right after her honeymoon. We had a lot of training to do. Training anyone for this job is a monumental task. She had to learn every aspect of the spa in order to know how to manage it. Soon after starting, she told me she was pregnant. Her due date was thirty-eight weeks from her start date: a honeymoon baby. We were all thrilled for her. She promised that she would continue to work full-time after her maternity leave. She had so much enthusiasm for the business. I spent the next eight months training her. Some things she took to well. Others were painful. It turned out she had no affinity for phone etiquette. She just did not make people feel like she cared about them and seemed dismissive. One of the things that sets us apart is that we will go the extra mile for our patients. Whatever you need, we will figure it out. Penny sounded like she couldn't care less. Other areas that I had hoped she would manage, she never took to. Payroll, numbers, tracking, incentives. However, she was really great at Instagram.

For eight months, we made slow progress. As it got closer to her due date, I made plans for resuming the process when she got back. She took four months off for maternity leave. I was willing to give her however long she wanted, as long as she was coming back. She promised she would. In those four months, I went back to doing the few things she had taken over, except Instagram—I was still lousy at that. But I found that the total time it took me to do my job and hers was minimally more than I had been spending when she was on the payroll. Nonetheless, I was looking forward to having her back in her role and to continue to delegate more responsibilities to her. Days before she was to return, she quit.

The few times people have left my spa, I have felt it was the right thing in the end. My efforts to make it work are not always worth it. Sometimes it is just not meant to be. I felt this way with Penny just as much as I did with RN#2. I have a tendency to try to make things work, like in a bad marriage. I have learned a lot from owning a business. Now for every new hire, I not only have a comprehensive job description but also have a success checklist that we review at ninety days to make sure the employee is on track. It does not help the business or employee to have a job drag on if it is the wrong one.

KEY TAKEAWAYS

FROM THIS CHAPTER

1. Persistence and Believing in Yourself: I was laughed at by my old radiology group when I proposed starting an aesthetic practice. Instead of being discouraged, I was energized. I took matters into my own hands, securing a location, insurance, and a domain for the business. Believe in yourself and your ideas, even when others may doubt you.

2. Find the Right People: My experience trying to find the right manager for my spa is a lesson for any business owner, about the need to have people who align with your business values and can help you achieve your vision.

3. If you have a bad experience on the phone or in person at a place you've loved before, tell the manager or owner! They really want to know. If it is a great place, they will fix it, give further training, and whatever it takes.

CHAPTER 9

AESTHETIC PROCEDURES MADE SIMPLE

I n this chapter, I explain the basics of the most common aesthetic procedures and why they sometimes go so terribly wrong. By the end of the chapter, you'll know exactly what to look for if you're in the market for any of these, and you'll know what to ask to ensure you're getting the best service.

WHY BOTOX® IS LIKE CRACK (IN A GOOD WAY!)

When I say Botox®, what I really mean is any of the neurotoxins we use for cosmetic purposes. Botox® has become a generic word for cosmetic neurotoxin. It is much easier to say, right? A lot of the time I just say "toxin" to refer to any of them. In the United States, there are five neurotoxins that are currently FDA-approved. Botox® was the first, but now there are many competitors. Dysport® is the biggest competitor in part because most unbiased observers find that it acts quicker and lasts longer than Botox®. Xeomin® is a third toxin that is sold as though it is equivalent to Botox®, but most people find it doesn't last as long. The new kids on the block are Jeuveau® and

Daxxi®. There is less data on Jeuveau®, but most people seem to think it also does not last quite as long as Botox®. Daxxi® is the newest, and they claim it lasts up to 50 percent longer than Botox®. Since its launch, Daxxi® has been found by most doctors not to last longer than Botox®, and the stock price of the company that makes it has plummeted. For the purposes of this chapter, I'm going to refer to all of these as "toxin."

WHAT DOES TOXIN DO?

Toxins block the transmission of signal from the nerve ending to the muscle. The muscle is then paralyzed, so the wrinkles it causes go away. The most common place we put toxin is the glabella—the place between your eyebrows where you get those deep vertical lines—the 11's. I love to treat this area, because when the glabella is paralyzed, you can no longer make the mean angry face. The only thing this facial expression conveys is anger or concern. If you draw a stick figure with an angry face, the two diagonal lines above the eyes are the corrugator muscles. There is also a vertical one between the corrugators called the

procerus. Together, these muscles make those deep wrinkles that so many of us wear almost constantly. When you treat those people, they look kinder, nicer, happier, less stressed, and younger. A nice side effect is that headaches decrease or go away entirely. The first time you do it, people will ask you where you just went on vacation. Or they'll say you look relaxed or happy. Or in my case, they said, "Kate, you look less angry." Boy, that made me mad! Did I always look angry before? Apparently I did.

You can also treat crow's feet. Those are the crinkles at the side of your eyes. When we treat them, they pretty much disappear.

We start to get these in our twenties, but they progress quite a bit. If you look at Hugh Grant, you'll see his crow's feet have taken over his entire face. I'm a huge Hugh Grant fan. And he's a great example of how men can wear their wrinkles and be called "distinguished," whereas women with the same lines are "haggard." The double standard is in large part why we are busy getting rid of these wrinkles with toxin.

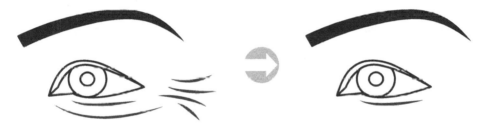

Toxins are also commonly used to treat the forehead lines. Those are the horizontal lines that stretch clear across your forehead when you make a surprised expression. Many people say "forehead" when they really mean the glabella. In general, it is often best to treat both at the same time for an even natural look. But they can be treated alone as well—it can just be tricky. The forehead muscles are always pulling up on the eyebrows. When you treat them, the eyebrow can change their shape and can lower. Sometimes, this will happen more on one side than the other. This doesn't mean the person who did the injections necessarily injected more on one side—because those muscles are so very often asymmetric themselves—they may actually need to be treated more on one side than the other. The forehead can be the trickiest area to treat with toxin because of those pesky brows. For this reason, I try to explain exactly how it works and what I'm trying to do so that people understand just what they are asking for.

There are many other places we can use toxin, though only certain toxins are approved for certain things. Physicians can use drugs and medical devices off-label if they choose, so long as they are well founded in their use as far as safety and effectiveness. So the glabella, crow's feet, and forehead are the big three. But there are a number of other things we can do with toxins.

Brow Lift: A small amount of toxins in the orbicularis oculi muscle (which pulls down on the eyebrow) will allow the frontalis (forehead muscle) to tug the brow up slightly. This will give a subtle 2–3 millimeter lift to the brow. For people with heavy lids or flat eyebrows, this can be beautiful. But remember it requires the frontalis to *move*. That means you can't always get rid of all forehead wrinkles and *also* get a brow lift. It is a delicate balance and an art.

Resting Bitch Face (RBF): The corners of the mouth often turn down and create a permanent frown. A tiny amount of toxins in the depressor anguli oris (DAO) muscle will stop that tugging and allow the corners to even out. Too much and you look like the Joker. A bit in the wrong spot, and you can get an uneven smile. Again, it is a delicate balance and an art.

Dimpled Chin: Some people have an orange peel or dimpled look to the chin. A tiny bit in the mentalis can eliminate that. A bit in the wrong place can give you an uneven lower lip. It is an art, people! Things can go wrong.

Teeth Grinding: Toxins injected in the masseters (jaw muscles) can stop teeth grinding and clenching. A little bit too high and you can get an uneven smile. Yikes!

Bunny Lines: A tiny bit in the upper nose and those bunny lines disappear. I have actually not ever seen a complication from this, but I'm sure it could happen.

Lip Lines: A tiny amount in the upper lip can reduce the lip lines (or smoker's lines—though many people have them who don't smoke). This is also a very delicate area, because too much and you can't take a sip of tea without dribbling. And try kissing! It can get dicey.

Notice that I keep repeating "a tiny bit." Well, we are talking about the lower face. You need your lower face to talk and smile and eat. We simply can't mess with that too much. The lower face really needs different kinds of attention rather than just throwing Botox® at the problem. If you do too much, you just look frozen. We really need to talk about other options.

What happens when Botox® goes wrong? Droopy eyebrows, droopy eyelids, asymmetric smile, Joker face, and Dr. Spock eyebrows. Sometimes even weirder. Injecting Botox® is an art.

OVERSTUFFED SYNDROME: THE SCOOP ON DERMAL FILLERS

Why do so many people suffer from overstuffed syndrome?

So many people are terrified of fillers. They've seen the Hollywood stars looking bizarre, and they've seen their friends puffy and weird. Why do people end up looking overstuffed and stiff?

I will never give someone ducky lips. I simply do not believe that ducky lips make people look beautiful. How is it that we see more and more people looking overstuffed with fillers? Giant ducky lips, huge cheeks, a lower face that doesn't really move when they talk. These things do not look natural and often are so distracting, one spends more time thinking about why this person looks so odd than listening to what they are saying. So why does this happen?

As you age, you lose volume in your face. When we are kids, we have fat pads that round out the face and give us a baby-face look. As you get older, you lose those fat pads over time. Eventually, you get hollows and areas that look scooped out. Fillers are one solution that can help replace volume. And when done well, they can really make you look younger. Fillers are a great tool, but they are not the only tool.

The big process that contributes just as much to aging is the thinning of the skin. After around age thirty, the cells in your dermis that make collagen and elastin go dormant. Your body breaks those down at 1–2 percent per year, so after that, your skin is slowly thinning out. As it thins, it is no longer thick and springy, and it starts to sag. Here's the problem: many injectors use fillers to prop up this sagging skin. They put volume in until the skin is taut. It is like adding a few tent poles under stretched-out tent fabric. If they put enough filler in, you start to look like a balloon. The results can be dramatic, and they are instant (although temporary). But what happens over time as your skin continues to thin out? You need more and more filler to prop it up.

Dermal fillers can be a great option for cheeks and the hollows under the eyes. They can also be used to soften the lines of the lower face, if used judiciously. But since the problem is largely that the skin is too stretched out and lax, the lower face is usually wrinkly because skin from the upper face is hanging down. What you need is often lift, not yet more volume in the lower face. Adding too much filler into the lower face can make a person look very abnormal. Small amounts of a flexible filler in strategic areas can look great. Larger amounts make the lower face look uncomfortably swollen and bizarre.

If the only tool you have is filler, you end up chasing this increasing problem of sagging skin with more and more filler. Eventually, you look ridiculous, and you still have not addressed the real problem—a loss of collagen and thinning skin. Places that do not offer other tools, or have an approach more focused on creating repeat filler customers, are missing the opportunity to address the whole problem, and they are overstuffing people in the process. Many injectors are paid more if they inject more, and they may not want to refer patients for skin tightening if they don't offer that or if they do but the injector won't make money from it. Financial incentives often motivate injectors to do more.

The best practice is to use a combination of approaches to tighten skin and replace volume that makes you look like you, just a bit younger. Filler is always an option—it is a great tool! But we also focus on building your collagen with tools like microneedling with RF, laser resurfacing, PRP and microneedling, and Sculptra®, a non-filler injectable that also builds collagen. There is also a device called Emface, which induces collagen and also stimulates the lifting muscles of the face, lifting the lower face and increasing the cheek volume without fillers. Taking great care of your skin is also critical to keep it looking young and healthy. Most importantly, we are looking at the big picture and using our resources for the long term.

For an up-to-date list of filler recommendations, see the online content at medspamayhem.com.

Questions to ask before having filler:

- How much of my problem is volume loss, and how much is loose skin?

    □ If I have loose skin, do you have options for skin tightening?

- What kind of filler are you using? (Hyaluronic acid fillers versus others)

- How much will I need, and what are the alternatives?

- Can you make sure I don't end up looking like a balloon?

PRESERVING YOUTHFUL SKIN AND APPEARANCE WITHOUT LOOKING WEIRD

MAINTAIN AND REBUILD COLLAGEN

Here's the most important thing I have to share with you: keep your fibroblasts awake!

Why does the skin thin out and lose elasticity as you age? By the time you turn thirty, the cells in your skin that make collagen and elastin go dormant. Collagen and elastin are what keep your skin thick and springy—and resistant to gravity. And the fibroblasts that make them fall asleep and *stop* making it. By age thirty! And your body breaks them down at about 1–2 percent per year. So, for the rest of your adult life, the skin is thinning out. Often, by age eighty, the skin is completely see-through. That's because the dermis is gone.

This is why we suddenly notice in our late thirties or early forties that our skin just does not look the same. It almost feels like it happened overnight. But, in fact, by that time, it has been going on for a decade or more. You just don't notice in the beginning because when you've only lost a few percent, it is hard to detect. One day after so many years, something will trigger you to take a closer look in the mirror. Maybe you have a new sunspot or wrinkle or zit. Maybe you just got Botox® for the first time. Something gets you to take a deeper look and you realize you don't quite look like your twenty-six-year-old self anymore.

This is why it is so important—to *keep your fibroblasts awake*! This is totally possible. There are several easy treatments that poke at your fibroblasts and wake them up and stimulate collagen. Each time, the fibroblasts respond with around four to six months of collagen, and then they peter out. So the idea is to poke at them every three to four months to keep them awake and productive all year. You must at least make up for the 1–2 percent loss. That will preserve the thick, springy skin you already have. If your skin is already thin and starting to fall, you need more powerful treatments to thicken and tighten the skin. These treatments range in cost, benefits, and downtime.

I believe that preserving your natural beauty by maintaining collagen is a long-term preventive approach to aging. It is much easier to prevent thinning than to tighten later. If you are in your thirties, it is great to start now before you have lost much of the elements that keep your face youthful.

What are the options for maintaining collagen, and which ones work the best? For a detailed up-to-date list of options, check our website at medspa-insider.com.

WHEN TO USE DERMAL FILLER

Dermal filler is a fantastic tool to restore facial volume that has been lost with aging. It can be used to fill the hollows under the eyes and cheeks. It can also be used to fill very fine lines of the surface of the skin and, of course, restore volume to the lips. Fillers can be used to strengthen the jawline and chin. The idea is to replace what has been lost and not to overfill. This can be tricky when your financial incentive is to do more, not less. I described Overstuffed Syndrome in the previous section. That should be avoided. But dermal fillers can play an important role in decreasing wrinkles. Early studies of the first filler, Restylane®, found that the body makes its own collagen in areas where the filler has been injected so that even long after the filler has dissolved, it has some long-lasting anti-wrinkle effects.

There are certain areas where fillers are the only option to fill volume loss. Under the eyes (the tear trough) is a spot where you cannot place any other product safely (though PRP and platelet-rich fibrin matrix [PRFM] are an option here, just a bit more expensive). Fillers are also the ideal choice to precisely contour the cheeks and jawline, though Sculptra® can help with these as well.

FILLER ALTERNATIVES

Sculptra Aesthetic® is an injectable that many people confuse with fillers. It comes as a powder and is reconstituted in sterile water. When injected into the skin and just beneath the skin, it stimulates the body's own natural collagen to build up. Sculptra® is a powdered form of poly-L-lactic acid (PLLA). PLLA has been used in absorbable stitches for many years. It causes a collagen buildup and then dissolves. The collagen that is created by your body is long-lasting and will break down with the aging process as the rest of your collagen does—at about 1–2 percent per year. The effect of Sculptra® takes months to develop and can continue to improve over one to two years after injection. Then the results are fairly long-lasting.

Sculptra® was initially developed in the 1990s to treat facial wasting associated with HIV/AIDS. It worked so well that it was co-opted by the aesthetic industry for facial rejuvenation. Sculptra® is a great tool for people who have lost a lot of volume in the face. It can be used to augment cheeks and the lower face, softening the nasolabial folds and marionette lines, leading to a rounder, smoother appearance.

Initially, when Sculptra® was FDA approved, it was diluted in a small amount of saline. The treatment worked well, but sometimes, patients would develop firm nodules under the skin. These nodules were not treatable except by surgical excision. Many dermatologists and plastic surgeons abandoned it at the time because of nodules. But over the last couple of decades, techniques have changed. Sculptra® is now diluted with twice the amount of water that was used in the '90s. The result is that we rarely, if ever, see nodules anymore. There are some who will still not use Sculptra® because of this risk, but I have found it to be incredibly consistent and have yet to see a single nodule in my practice. Sculptra® maintains an important role in restoring youthful skin because it works so well and has such long-lasting results.

THE SKINNY ON BODY SCULPTING

BODY SCULPTING DEVICES

In the past, the only options for getting rid of stubborn unwanted fat was with surgery or liposuction. That required general anesthesia, scarring, risk of infection, and lots of downtime. In the last fifteen years, there has been a revolution in technology that removes fat without surgery or downtime. It turns out that you can freeze fat, heat fat, and even blast it with high-intensity ultrasound, and fat cells actually die, and the fat inside them is excreted by your body. Technology has come a long way since the old machines that merely jiggle your fat.

The first technology that really worked to kill fat was freezing—with CoolSculpting®. This machine has been around since 2010 and uses plastic applicator cups to vacuum fat and freeze it. Details about

CoolSculpting® were discussed in chapter 7. As a reminder, CoolSculpting® really works to kill fat, but it has some limitations. Patient selection is super important to get the best results, and the big issue is that we don't really know how common a complication called paradoxical hyperplasia really is.

Competitors to CoolSculpting® have used RF, ultrasound, and lasers to heat the skin and the fat from the skin surface—to tighten the skin and kill the fat. Many devices have been invented for this, each with middling results.

Then BTL invented Emsculpt and then Emsculpt Neo. It uses magnetic waves that cause supramaximal contractions of the muscle. Supramaximal means that these contractions are way more than what you would normally do in any vigorous workout. These contractions are more powerful than your brain can make your muscle do. Emsculpt does this about 20,000 times in a half-hour treatment. Though intense, it doesn't hurt. The result is a stronger, more sculpted muscle. In the studies done to validate Emsculpt, it was found to kill fat as well. Emsculpt Neo added RF heating to maximize results. There have been seven published studies of the Emsculpt Neo. The results showed marked increase in muscle mass and decrease in fat on MRI, CT, and ultrasound. On average, there was a 25 percent increase in muscle and a 30 percent decrease in fat one month after a series of treatments.

Emsculpt Neo is currently FDA-cleared to treat the abdomen, love handles, buttocks, thighs, arms (biceps and triceps), and calves. The Emsculpt Neo protocol is a series of four thirty-minute treatments. The big advantage of Emsculpt Neo over CoolSculpting® is that there is almost no risk of complications, like PAH. Plus the vast majority of patients feel it gives good results. A win-win.

With the advent of GLP-1 drugs (like Ozempic® or semaglutide), many people are choosing this medical treatment to lose weight. The use of body sculpting devices has decreased as a result. But it turns out Emsculpt Neo and Emface might very well be surging next—because people who have lost the weight on semaglutide end up with "O" Body and "O Face," and they look better after building muscle and tightening skin.

For the latest recommendation on body sculpting, see our website at medspamayhem.com.

CELLULITE

Why is it so hard to get rid of cellulite? Over the years, I have seen many treatments that claim to reduce or even eliminate cellulite. However, I've never seen a treatment that actually works well. There are some treatments that can give a temporary improvement, and if you look at those before and after pictures, it can be very convincing. But the results are fleeting. In this section, I'll explain what cellulite is and why it is so tough, what we can do for body sculpting, and what the limitations are.

What Is Cellulite?

Cellulite is mostly seen around the thighs but can happen elsewhere in the body. It consists of fatty areas that have dimpling of the skin surface. The result is a wavy, dimpled, fatty appearance. The dimples happen because the fat around the thighs is permeated with fibrous bands of connective tissue, much like a honeycomb. The thighs have this structure that is very different from other parts of your body, like your belly. Imagine the belly fat as a tub of butter. You could take a spoon and scoop it all out. Now imagine that the thigh fat is like a honeycomb with fat in each little pocket. If you tried to scoop that out, you wouldn't get much—you would be blocked by a band of tissue. Now imagine you add butter to each space. The belly just expands and fills up. But the thighs, those fibrous bands are attached to the skin. As you add fat, the skin bulges out, but the attachments to the skin are tugged in, resulting in a dimple. This is why cellulite looks like it does.

Treatments for Cellulite

Thigh Creams: No matter what is in a cream, there is no way it is going to penetrate through your skin and release those bands or kill fat. Save your money.

Shock Wave: There are several devices that send shock waves into the tissue in an attempt to loosen the bands. Experiments using shock waves to loosen and smooth out cellulite can show minimal temporary improvement, but this is short-lived and not enough to throw money at it. There are many devices out there that purport to do this—don't waste your money.

Cellfina®: This is a semi-invasive procedure that uses a device to target individual dimples in the skin, and the physician slices through the band through the skin surface. Cellfina® can really produce some nice results. But they are temporary. Why? If you are going in there and literally cutting the band, why would the results be temporary? Because (unfortunately) the bands re-tether over time. That's right—your body rebuilds those bands as it heals. The dimples return. Plus it is fairly invasive and expensive. This procedure was exciting when it first came out, but you'll find few places offering it now.

Surgery and liposuction: Believe it or not, surgery doesn't work much better than Cellfina® for the same reasons. If you take a scalpel and slice through one of those cellulite bands—it just re-tethers! As a matter of fact, those fibrous bands are really difficult to deal with during liposuction as well. Let's go back to that tub of butter. With liposuction, you are using a vacuum to suck out the fat. The belly (and some other areas) are ideal for this, and results can be beautiful. But the thighs, they bump into those bands and can't get through them or lyse (to burst or cut a cell or cell structure) through some but not others. The results of liposuction on the thighs are often weirdly lumpy and wavy. The bands make it so that you have to cut into each tiny pocket of fat to vacuum it out—and this is really challenging.

Injectables: There was an injectable medication called Qwo that was sold for cellulite treatment. It went off the market after about a year. There were only two studies of Qwo with only a few patients in each. They showed a 6 percent and 9 percent significant improvement that both the patient and the doctor could agree upon. They showed a 50 percent minimal improvement that either the doctor or the patient felt was present, but others disagreed. The one-year follow-up showed a 34 percent overall long-term success rate. Meanwhile, the treatment causes massive, dark bruising that can cover the entirety of the patient's legs and thighs. Long term with that much bruising, the body is often left with hemosiderin deposits that can permanently stain the skin.

With a low success rate and terrible bruising like this, the product did not do well.

Body Sculpting—What Can We Really Do for Cellulite?

There are three big things we *can* do with our machines. We can kill fat, we can build muscle, and we can tighten skin. We cannot dissolve those bands! At least not very effectively with long-lasting results, and that is what I'm looking for. Treatment for thighs can result in a significant improvement in the appearance of fat and cellulite. If you reduce the fat and build muscle, the cellulite will look better since there is less fat bulging out, thus less tugging in of the skin. The thighs are large areas and have four muscle groups (the quads in front, buttocks and hamstrings in back, and the adductors on the inner thigh and abductors on the outer thighs). That's a lot of treatments. It is definitely not a one-and-done magical cellulite vanishing cream. I wish I could invent that!

Cellulite is one of the most challenging issues we try to address in aesthetic medicine. The fibrous bands that cause the dimpling appearance are really strong, resistant to any kind of treatment, and have a very strong tendency to recur. The best treatments focus on the realistic goals of reducing fat, toning muscle, and improving skin.

OZEMPIC® (SEMAGLUTIDE) AND GLP1-AGONISTS

Ozempic® is a drug developed for diabetes that has taken the weight-loss industry by storm—and in its wake, med spas all over the country are cashing in. The drugs themselves are dramatically successful at inducing weight loss but carry with them many side effects, some of which are very harmful. These drugs mimic the effects of the hormone in your body that makes you feel full and sated. They can help you lose a ton of weight, if used carefully and if you are lucky enough not to suffer too many of the side effects, which can include nausea, diarrhea, pancreatitis, pain, hypoglycemia, dizziness, thyroid problems, and even thyroid cancer.

The demand for these drugs has way outstripped the ability of the maker of Ozempic® (Novo Nordisk) to make enough of it. As a result, compounding pharmacies have been given the legal ability to make generic forms of it under an "emergency order." Pharmacies all over the country are busy making as much as they can to meet the supply. While many of these pharmacies are doing so legally, many are illegally making different forms of the drug that are *not* FDA-approved. These drugs can be directly purchased online by anyone who will click a box saying that they are using it only for research purposes. Unscrupulous people have easy access, getting the drugs online without a doctor's license and turning around and selling it directly to patients for injection.

Beware of any business offering semaglutide for medical weight loss—they may be using unapproved forms of the drug and may be offering it without physician oversight. These drugs must be prescribed by a physician with careful monitoring. They are instead being purchased and distributed illegally by people who just want a piece of the action. Always ask to see a doctor first. Ask who is prescribing the drug, where does it come from, and what form of the drug it is and is it FDA-approved.

WHY IS LASER HAIR REMOVAL SO EXPENSIVE?

For many years, there was a Groupon every day for laser hair removal. It was super cheap. There were several laser chain businesses that always ran Groupons, and it was impossible to compete with that. There are many different kinds of lasers that can be used for this. The best ones are very expensive (should I buy a house or a laser?). The top lasers for hair removal have two lasers in one: Alexandrite (to treat lighter skin) and Nd-Yag (to treat darker skin). There are also diode lasers that are OK at removing hair but less safe for darker skin types. Then there are IPL devices that are effective on lighter skin only and tend to be pretty slow. IPL is great for lots of things but clunky and slow for laser hair removal.

It was hard to understand how any business could offer the service at such a low price, much less split that with Groupon. But they did. I couldn't compete, so I decided I would not be doing it in my office. I had an IPL device early on, so I could offer the service. But there was no way I could compete on price. And it was slow, so I couldn't compete on speed either. We did not do a lot of laser hair removal.

Then several bankruptcies happened. American Laser filed Chapter 11 in 2014 and LightRx in 2019. Many individual spas that did laser hair removal went out of business as well. The Groupons went away. Prices rose. Why is it so expensive? The true cost of laser hair removal reflects not only the cost of the device itself and its maintenance (Alexandrite and Nd-Yag lasers have very expensive maintenance costs). It also costs a lot to pay a highly qualified person to perform the service. And then there is insurance. Overall, it is a pretty expensive service to offer. Once the chains went bankrupt that were somehow cutting corners to keep prices artificially low, the market price went back up to what it truly costs.

During the Covid-19 pandemic, the demand for laser hair removal in our spa skyrocketed. We saw a lot of people turn to self-care as a salve to our isolation and lack of other sources of joy and pleasure. Some people wanted to do their entire body. As the demand went up, we decided to invest in the top-of-the-line Alex/Yag laser—the fastest one in the industry. This wouldn't have been possible in the old Groupon days. If you are looking for a great place for laser hair removal, always keep in mind that lasers are not equal, just as providers of these services are not equal. Ask what laser they are using. If they give you a trade name, ask what type of laser it is. Find out who provides the service. Any time you use a laser, you risk getting burned. Burns should be a super-rare occurrence, but an experienced provider will be able to adjust settings to maximize your treatment while minimizing risk.

Questions to ask the spa if you are interested in having laser hair removal:

1. What kind of laser do you use?

2. Can you treat all types of skin? Ask about your skin type.

3. Who performs the service? How much experience do they have?

Any place you go to should perform an initial consultation by a doctor (or NP or PA). If they book you directly for the laser service, they are not operating legally.

SETTING EXPECTATIONS

Everything in aesthetics is about managing expectations. Well, let's face it—all of life is about managing expectations. That's why we spend so much time in our consultations explaining the science and expected outcomes, as well as possible pitfalls. That is also why I offer unlimited follow-up consultations for our existing patients so that we can have an ongoing open communication about how our treatments are working and what to expect. I truly feel that if you understand what the process is like, how you'll feel during and after, what to expect in recovery, and what kinds of outcomes we see, you'll have a much better experience. It is best if there are no surprises. If you have unrealistic expectations, we won't proceed.

There Is No Magic Body: A large man with a big belly came in for a consultation for body sculpting. His belly was starting to interfere with the steering wheel while driving, and he was hoping for help. He had high blood pressure, diabetes, and poor diet and did not exercise. When we talked to him about our body sculpting program, we explained that it is not a weight loss program and machines are not a substitute for a proper diet and exercise. In order to have a worthwhile investment, you would have to comply with basic health recommendations. He looked at the product display on our wall and asked, "Don't you just have a cream I can use?" Unfortunately, no.

I Can't Make You Look Like Angelina Jolie: Probably, the most common star people would like to emulate is Angelina. And no matter what the angle, no, I cannot make your jaw or cheekbones look like hers.

Kylie Jenner Lips: Yes, we can plump your lips. But no, we cannot make you look like Kylie. Just so you know, Kylie stopped making them that big a long time ago now.

The Perfect Jawline: One young woman walked into the spa asking for fillers for the jawline. She saw one of our providers who explained how fillers work and what we can do and what we can't. She was upset. She came in with a picture of someone who didn't look anything like her and said she wanted that jawline. Now, fillers can be used to augment the jawline. But it takes a lot of filler, and it doesn't last. And despite what you might have seen on Instagram, you can't just magically look like someone else.

Part of our job is to help people see their own natural beauty. We can help you look your best. But anyone telling you they can make you look like someone else—without surgery—well, they are selling you a fantasy. And they are going to charge you a premium. When the provider came out of the room and asked for a second opinion, I went in to make my own assessment. This girl was beautiful. And she was teary. She didn't see herself as beautiful, and she thought if she looked like this model in the photo, somehow life would be better. So much of what we do is to reassure and shape expectations. It is best to let someone down a bit than to embark on an impossible fantasy. We hope we are doing it in a gentle and positive way.

THINGS TO WATCH OUT FOR:

If someone is promising you they can make you look like a model or celebrity, walk out the door.

If someone is setting realistic expectations, pay attention. They are telling you the truth.

THE STEM CELL MYTHS

Back in 2012, *60 Minutes* did a story on an Alabama physician named Dan Ecklund, who had lost his US medical license in 2005 for having prescribed controlled substances to a patient with whom he was having sex and for having admitted to having sex with underage girls. He then founded a stem cell company based in Ecuador that shipped supposed "human stem cells" to the United States. He was a supposed "self-taught" expert, who decided to manufacture stem cells in his own lab. He sold these stem cells to desperate patients who had permanent deficits that had no treatment for many thousands of dollars. The story was so egregious, you might think this wouldn't happen in the United States, right?

There are many medical spas in the country that have expanded into the stem cell scam. They are touted as a miracle treatment, being used for all manner of diseases, whether or not they have legitimate mainstream treatments.

In Seattle, there was a med spa owned by Dr. Tami. In 2018, Dr. Tami founded a stem cell company called US Stemology. You might remember Dr. Tami from an earlier chapter. She is the one who calls herself double board certified despite having not even completed a residency. She sold this unproven stem cell treatment to people who had nowhere else to turn. In an exposé on a local TV news station, one young man who was paralyzed from a spinal cord injury was interviewed with his family. They believed the treatment would work, even though he regained none of his function. The stem cells being sold were supposedly harvested from umbilical cords. Then in 2020, as the pandemic ensued, US Stemology sold the treatment as a cure for Covid-19. She treated a total of 107 patients for over $750,000, as charged by the attorney general, who sued her in 2022.[15] Her business was ultimately shut down, and she had to pay a $500,000 fine. She had to offer refunds to all 107 patients.

A very similar case unfolded in 2021 in New York, involving Dr. Joel Singer and his clinic Park Avenue Stem Cell.[16] This one resulted in an over $5 million settlement.

This kind of scam is happening all around the United States. Stem cells from fetal tissue have long been promised as a possible solution to many untreatable diseases. The hope is that pluripotent cells (cells that have the ability to become any type of cell) could grow into brain cells (in the case of stroke or Alzheimer's patients) or heart cells for people with heart damage. There are ongoing research efforts to figure out if this is possible, and if so, how to do it. But we have not succeeded yet. The science is simply not there.

What about stem cells from the bone marrow? Yes, we have been using those for bone marrow transplants for many years now. These cells have the ability to grow new bone marrow, so the idea is that we isolate bone marrow stem cells, give radiation to kill a cancer, and

---

15   "AG Ferguson wins $500,000 for individuals impacted by US Stemology's unproven claims that its stem cell injections could treat COVID-19 and other medical conditions," https://www.atg.wa.gov/news/news-releases/ag-ferguson-wins-500000-individuals-impacted-us-stemology-s-unproven-claims-its.

16   New York State Attorney General, "Attorney General James secures $5.1 million judgment against New York city stem cell clinic for scamming patients out of thousands through false advertising," https://ag.ny.gov/press-release/2021/attorney-general-james-secures-51-million-judgment-against-new-york-city-stem.

then regrow the bone marrow. You need bone marrow to live because that is what makes red blood cells (your blood) and white blood cells (your immunity). But can stem cells from the bone marrow grow into brain cells or heart cells? No, they cannot.

What about "stem cells" from the fat? Can they do anything for you? The short answer is no. Not now. Science does not have this ability.

If you are interested in the topic, there is a fantastic and compelling podcast about the stem cell industry gone bad, called "Bad Batch," by Wondery.[17] I highly recommend it. The *60 Minutes* story[18] is entertaining as well, and they ambush the doctor.

Take-Home Message: Stem Cell Clinics Are a Scam. Just Don't Go.

PLATELET-RICH PLASMA (PRP) AND PLATELET-RICH FIBRIN MATRIX (PRFM)

An example of Off-Label Use is the use of Platelet-Rich Plasma or PRP for all manner of medical procedures. PRP is a product produced from the patient's own blood. It is therefore a blood product, and its injection is not regulated by the FDA. PRP was used experimentally for various musculoskeletal problems in the 1970s and continued to be developed for new uses over the next several decades. It wasn't until 2009 that the first system of blood collection and centrifugation was FDA-approved to produce PRP. After that, many other systems have

---

17   "Bad batch," https://wondery.com/shows/bad-batch/.

18   CBS News, "Stem cell fraud: a 60 minutes investigation," https://www.cbsnews.com/news/stem-cell-fraud-a-60-minutes-investigation-26-08-2012/.

been cleared through the 510(k) process. What doctors do with the PRP is not regulated. Doctors have tried it for almost everything.

When I started in aesthetics in 2014, PRP for facial rejuvenation was taught in one of the advanced courses I attended. The idea is that PRP has very potent growth factors that rejuvenate the skin by stimulating new collagen and elastin. This makes logical sense. The procedure involved direct injections of PRP into hard-to-treat critical areas, using it with microneedling to spread these growth factors throughout the skin. Although there are no real studies proving it worked, Kim Kardashian had posted about her Vampire Facial®, and before you knew it, everyone wanted one. It is especially appealing because these are your own natural growth factors, and you are using a part of your own biology to stimulate the rejuvenation process. The cost to begin providing these procedures was minimal. I decided to give it a try.

The Vampire Facial® and Vampire Facelift® are procedures trademarked by Charles Runels, MD. Dr. Runels is board certified in internal medicine and practiced emergency medicine before migrating to aesthetic medicine. The terms are trademarked, and Dr. Runels charges a monthly fee for a practitioner to be certified and to allow them to use the terminology in advertising. However, the procedures using PRP, microneedling, and dermal fillers are ones done by physicians every day.

My first few patients specifically sought me out because not very many providers were doing PRP facial rejuvenation yet, and they wanted to try the procedure. It was hard to say what it would do ahead of time, but these first few people had done their own research and just wanted to try it. I made no promises. After years of experience I can say that it helps, but it is not a facelift. The procedure can definitely smooth out some of the very fine lines and wrinkles if done in a series of three or more. It can definitely decrease active acne and reduce pore size. And it builds enough collagen to prevent loss. So if you did around three procedures a year, you can stave off the thinning out that happens over time, preventing further drooping of the skin. But if you are looking for skin tightening, PRP will not be enough.

Do we have studies showing that what I just described is true? No, we do not.

Very soon after I started providing PRP facial rejuvenation, a fifty-two-year-old African American nurse midwife came for a consultation. Jaqueline (not her real name) had pronounced androgenic alopecia (male-pattern baldness), which is very common among women. She had tried Rogaine without much effect. She had been researching PRP for hair loss for the last two years and had interviewed every provider in the Seattle area who offered PRP. I was her last stop. She wanted to try PRP for her hair loss, and she wanted me to do it. I told her I hadn't used PRP for this indication, and she told me to go home and do my research and let her know. She had made her decision.

I researched everything I could on PRP for hair loss. There were few sources of information that were credible. One blog I found followed a young woman who had tried everything for her alopecia following her journey through PRP treatment, which she said worked for her. There was one doctor (Joseph Greco) in Florida who had published his own data, stating at the time that 70 percent of his patients responded to PRP injections for hair loss. I watched videos of multiple different doctors performing the injections. It was technically not difficult, and I already had the equipment to do it.

From the research I did, it would take a series of treatments about four to six weeks apart and at least three to four months to see improvement with less loss and new hair growth. If it worked, then you'd have to keep doing the procedure around two to three times each year to maintain results or the hair would start falling out again. That seemed like a big commitment to me. I wasn't sure whether people would even be interested in something that you had to keep doing to maintain. I called Jaqueline and told her I'd give it a shot. I revealed the results of my research and made no guarantees. But if she was up for an experiment, I'd do it.

Jaqueline came in for a treatment. The first thing I learned is that it is hard to numb up the scalp. The hair is in the way of any topical anesthetic sinking into the scalp. The second thing was that other than that, the procedure was very easy to do. At the time, many providers were both injecting PRP into the scalp and doing microneedling over it. Since then, most providers have dropped the microneedling part. The procedure went smoothly, and Jaqueline went home.

About two months later, I got another call: it was working! Her stylist saw lots of new growth, and the new baby hairs were black, very visible on her mostly gray head. She was excited, as was I. To this day, those are the most dramatic before and after images I have for PRP. I knew this was just one person. But it was exciting for me to be able to help with a problem that doctors have no answers for.

Since that time, I have performed many procedures for hair loss. The procedure itself has evolved. We use activated PRP (or PRF— Platelet-Rich Fibrin) now, and we no longer do the microneedling part. I also recommend a hair-health supplement and topical alopecia prescription medication to support the PRP treatments. About 75 percent of those patients self-report improvement. Only about a third choose to continue maintenance. I've seen both men and women. Men see a response, but in my experience never continue into maintenance. At some point, they decide to just go bald, which they can do, because they are men. The women are much more motivated to continue treatment. Being bald is simply not an option.

I don't believe we will ever see any studies to prove that PRP is an effective treatment for hair loss. There are simply no financial incentives for the PRP companies to fund them. Because treatment of alopecia is generally not covered by insurance, those healthcare dollars are not available. I believe it will remain a fringe medical treatment.

For the latest info on the use of PRP in the treatment of hair loss, see our website at medspamayhem.com.

VAGINAL REJUVENATION: THE INSIDE STORY

I sat in a large auditorium at The Aesthetic Show, awaiting a live demonstration of vaginal rejuvenation using a new RF device. Behind a black curtain, a volunteer model was positioned with the handheld wand of the device entering her vagina and a video camera aimed to capture the show for all to see. This device was inserted in and out of her for twenty minutes in four quadrants. The master aesthetician who happened to be sitting next to me had just learned how to use this device and she was excited—it really works, she said. It tightens the tissue; it increases lubrication. It thickens the vaginal wall and decreases pain with intercourse. And it decreases dribbling! My first reaction was, really? Does it? And my second reaction was, I really do not want to get into the vagina business. But vaginal rejuvenation was the next big thing in aesthetics, and everyone was excited about it.

In medical school, I had loved OB/GYN. I had learned so much and felt so appreciated. Delivering babies was very rewarding, though I was never great at staying up all night to do it. Though I enjoyed it, OB/GYN was never my calling. When I saw what was happening with the rise of vaginal rejuvenation, I had to evaluate it, but I had no desire to move in that direction. The closest we came to the vagina was Brazilian laser hair removal. At least, we had experience in the general area. But I felt this should be left in the hands of specialists and surgeons. But that is not what happened.

There was so much hype and excitement, people started buying the devices, and soon almost every major aesthetic device company was competing in the market.

There are two different kinds of vaginal rejuvenation devices. The first was the Mona Lisa Touch. It is a CO_2 fractional laser—this is a similar technology to fractional lasers for the skin but used to resurface the vaginal wall. There are now many similar lasers for this purpose.

A second technology arose for the same purpose using RF. The first of these was called Thermi-Va®, but there are many more using this same technology as well. It was the Thermi-Va® I saw demonstrated at that big conference. Then every device company that already had RF technology made their own version and marketed them for vaginal rejuvenation.

DOES VAGINAL REJUVENATION WORK?

In a simple answer, yes. Both the laser and RF devices work well for their purpose with almost no downside. The vaginal wall tissue is stimulated, thickens, and makes more lubrication. The tissues are tightened, though usually this is temporary. Most patients report less (or eliminated) dribbling or urinary incontinence. And a better sex life. I have actually been surprised at how many people report an improved sex life. And with tighter tissues, even the husbands report being able to tell. I'm not making this up!

HOW I ENDED UP IN THE VAGINA BUSINESS

I had no intention of purchasing one of these devices. I felt strongly that most people seeking out this treatment were outside of our core customer base. Most people with urinary incontinence seek help from GYNs and urologists. These docs were unlikely to refer to a medical spa for treatment that was not covered by insurance. I didn't know how many people would seek treatment for dryness or pain, but I didn't think it was in my wheelhouse to help with that. And I just didn't want to get into the vagina business.

But, one day I got a call from my laser rep (the one guy I trust). My RF device was being upgraded. It had been called Exilis Elite— and we used it to tighten skin and kill fat back in the day. It was being reengineered to add ultrasound to improve the technology, and as part of the upgrade, it would now be able to do vaginal rejuvenation too. The new device was called Exilis Ultra. If I upgraded, I would get a new device with the new technology and a new warranty for a fairly low price. I called a special meeting of my staff. I presented the information and asked them, if we get this technology, will you be willing to do these procedures? I was surprised to hear from them, sure! They were already "down there" doing laser anyway. And they were all excited to try it themselves. After the meeting, I decided to go ahead with the upgrade. If it works, we'll use it. If it doesn't, at least we have a brand-new and improved machine.

I arranged a training session as soon as we got our new device. The vaginal treatment was called the "Ultra Femme 360." 360 was a reference to the circumferential RF in the probe—because it treats in a circle, the entire vaginal wall gets treated at the same time— and the inner treatment time was only eight minutes (compared to over twenty for the Thermi-Va®). We treated three women for free in exchange for a report on whether it worked for them—and what changed and what didn't. All three were thrilled. One reported that the dribbling she had after having babies was gone. One reported that everything felt tighter and she was pleased at the "appearance" of the outer tissues. And one called the next day to tell us, and I'm not making this up, that she had a giant orgasm in a position she had never been able to have one before. This is for real, I swear. So, now we all wanted to try it.

I personally had a small amount of dribbling after my twins were born. I had put up with this for thirteen years before treating with the Ultra Femme—and it resolved after three sessions. I've had many patients respond well for this same issue—mild dribbling responds pretty well. Those who deal with this (leaking just a bit when you run or do jumping jacks) are super happy to have any improvement that is so simple. Those with more severe incontinence may feel some improvement, but often the RF treatment is not enough for them. Most people do feel some tightening and improvement in lubrication. I have not asked about our patients' sexual pleasure, so I cannot report any real data on that.

THE FDA SLAMS THE DOOR ON THE VAGINA

Suddenly, after about a year and a half swimming along in a slow but steady stream of vaginas, the FDA shut it all down.[19] Why? There could have been a lot of burns maybe, but no. Actually there were no reports that I know of about vaginal burns. Overall the RF devices and even the laser devices had a great safety record. The answer: none of the devices had received FDA clearance for vaginal rejuvenation. These devices were *all* made with technology that had been cleared for other indications. But none of the companies had done any studies for vaginal rejuvena-

---

19   Sheila Kaplan, "Vaginal 'rejuvenation' treatments may be unsafe, the F.D.A. says," https://www.nytimes.com/2018/07/30/health/vaginal-laser-fda.html.

tion. They merely took existing technology and used it for another purpose with no studies, and marketed them accordingly. The FDA put the kibosh on the vagina business. The devices are still out there—the manufacturers just can't market them for the vagina.

Interestingly, there have since been many studies showing efficacy and safety of vaginal rejuvenation. A review in April 2021 in the journal *Dermatologic Surgery*,[20] evaluated fifty-nine studies and concluded, "This review demonstrates radiofrequency and laser are efficacious for the treatment of vaginal laxity and/or atrophy. Further research needs to be completed to determine which specific pathologies can be treated, if maintenance treatment is necessary, and long-term safety concerns."

YOU CANNOT SAY VAGINA ON FACEBOOK

One thing that will get you banned from Facebook is saying the word "vagina" or making any reference at all to women's intimate parts. Business pages that talk about it get banned. Many people in the industry use euphemisms like "Women's Intimate Wellness." This makes it a little bit hard to blog about. It is not like we are trying to post pictures! But really, we can't talk about it. Combine that with the FDA seal of disapproval, and you have a nonstarter. Which is sad, really. Because I truly believe it works! But I don't have the money to perform a study of my own (and face it—I left academics for a reason—just not my thing).

I'm truly hoping the academic world will do some big enough studies so that vaginal treatments with laser and RF become accepted. There is an awfully large number of women who would really benefit.

---

20   Margit L. W. Juhász, Dorota Z. Korta, Natasha Atanaskova Mesinkovska, "Vaginal Rejuvenation: A Retrospective Review of Lasers and Radiofrequency Devices," *Dermatologic Surgery* 47, no. 4 (2021):489–494, https://pubmed.ncbi.nlm.nih.gov/33165070/.

CHAPTER 10

LOOKING TOWARD THE FUTURE

WHAT IS LEGAL?

WHO CAN PRACTICE MEDICINE?

Just about everything we do at a medical spa is considered the practice of medicine. In the United States, you must have a license to practice medicine in order to practice medicine. In most states, that means you have to be a doctor. Just over half the states allow NPs to practice medicine independently, and five states allow PAs to do so as well, with some limits on the practice—and each state is different. That leaves a big question—can everyone else in the spa practice medicine on their own, legally? The answer is, no. So, if you go to a medical spa and have a medical service and never see a doctor (or an NP or a PA), that's illegal.

How is it that you can walk into a medical spa, see an RN for Botox®, and pay money for it? Can RNs do anything without working under a physician? No. Is this legal? No.

What about laser techs and aestheticians? Can they practice medicine? If you go to a med spa and get laser hair removal with a technician without seeing a doctor first, is that legal? No.

THE GOOD FAITH EXAM

What is supposed to happen is that as a new patient, you are seen by a doctor (or a PA or an NP in some states) for an initial consultation, where they perform an exam and formulate a plan for treatment. That physician can then either carry out that plan themselves or delegate part or all of the treatment to an RN or aesthetician who works under them, to carry out the treatment plan. This initial consultation is usually called a "good faith exam." A good faith exam cannot legally be performed by an RN or any other lower-level provider.

If the med spa does not have a doctor (or an NP or a PA) to perform a good faith exam, it is operating illegally. Many spas try to outsource this to a low-cost provider. There are services you can buy where an NP, often in another state, offers a virtual "good faith exam" by videoconference, so the spa can check this box. Unfortunately, it is very difficult to assess the skin and other conditions over video conference. And interestingly, it is very difficult to be licensed in every state in order to legally practice medicine this way. The services that offer a low-cost "good faith exam" may not be operating legally either, but it is a way for nonmedical providers to circumvent the law.

MEDICAL DIRECTORS

Every med spa must have a medical director. The medical director is an MD (or NP in some states) who is responsible for every medical procedure performed in the spa. The medical director is taking full liability for the procedure. If something goes wrong, it is their license on the line. All medical products and devices are purchased under their name. When you order Botox®, you must do so under the name of a doctor. All orders of things like Botox® are purchased under the medical director's name.

Many spas are owned and operated by a nonmedical owner. So they have to hire a medical director in order to do anything. Many of these spas do not want to pay a doctor's salary. So they search for an MD willing to act as a medical director at the lowest cost possible. The rate to rent a medical license is often as low as $500 to $1,000/month. They offer that as though it were free money. "We will list you on our books as medical director—and you don't have to do a thing!" Often, the medical director doesn't even work at the spa at all. There is often little or no oversight. But the spa can now purchase lasers and order Botox®, and they have their box checked: medical director, check.

I was interviewing an NP for a position in my practice who had been the medical director for another spa in my region for about a year. That spa is owned by an aesthetician and had a revolving door of medical directors. When I asked this NP about what she did for that spa, she said she never even worked there—was just listed as the medical director. When I asked her if she realized the liability she had taken on, she had no idea what she was doing. She was surprised and was thankful she wasn't doing it anymore. But let's be clear on what was happening: the med spa and the aesthetician who owned it were practicing medicine illegally under this NP's license, and the NP had no idea that what she was doing was so risky for her own license and what the med spa was doing was illegal. For the NP, it was a nice $1,000 each month that she didn't have to work for. She had no idea about the risks or consequences. Finally, she found out that long after she left there, they were still using her name to buy Botox®. Why? Because they still hadn't found a new medical director. That's right—they were no longer paying her to be the medical director but still had her name on their Botox® account. The NP only found this out when she tried to open her own Botox® account, and she was told her license was already being used by the spa. They were practicing medicine without a license *and* had no medical director. At least, until they convinced the next sucker to be their medical director. That revolving door keeps swinging around in circles.

OWNERSHIP: WHO CAN OWN A MEDICAL SPA?

We just answered the question, "Who can practice medicine?" But a related but different question is, "Who can own a medical practice?" The answer is similar but has even more far-reaching consequences. In almost every state, only a doctor can own a medical practice. These states have "Corporate Practice of Medicine," or CPOM, laws. These laws exist to protect patients and prevent a nondoctor from influencing the practice of medicine and preventing harm. That business has to be owned by a doctor (or NP in some states). Can it be solely owned by an aesthetician or RN or a businessperson? No. Can a nondoctor legally take payment for a medical service? No.

I am simplifying CPOM law here. I'm not a lawyer, and the laws are different in every state. I'm including this so that you can understand this: many med spas are illegally owned.

Some med spas are legally owned by nondoctors. How can that be possible?

There is a legal way. A businessperson can own a management services organization or MSO. That MSO can own a spa (not a med spa *or* a medical practice—but can own a spa). The MSO can lease space, hire personnel, buy skin and sell skin care products, schedule appointments, and so on. The MSO can form an agreement with a doctor to provide medical services within the spa. This agreement is called a "Management Services Agreement" or MSA. This agreement sets up the relationship between the doctor and the businessperson. The doctor must collect payment for the services provided, and the doctor must pay the MSO an agreed-upon fee. The flow of the money is important—from the patient to the doctor, who then pays the MSO.

Thus, for a businessperson to own a med spa, they must form an MSO and have an MSA in place with a doctor. Bank accounts must be separate, and the flow of money must be in the patient-to-doctor-to-MSO direction.

In a state that has a CPOM law, which includes the vast majority of the country, any spa owned by a nondoctor that does not have this setup is functioning illegally. If the spa is collecting the money into its account and then paying a medical director a monthly fee, that's illegal. If the spa has no MSA with the medical director, that's illegal. If the spa is not an MSO, that's illegal.

How many med spas across the United States function illegally? I honestly have no idea. I had no idea of the laws governing medical spas when I opened my own, and I doubt most spa owners do. The reason I know is that I joined the American Medical Spa Association (AmSpa) my first year in business, and legal compliance is one of their primary areas of focus. As I learned about these laws, I was grateful that what I was already doing was in compliance. Being an MD is a huge advantage in some ways. But it also costs much more to have an MD full-time on your staff. The places that cut out this expense can more easily offer services at lower prices. It creates a very uneven playing field—if you're illegally cutting costs you can compete on price—as long as you don't get caught.

WHO CAN INJECT BOTOX? CAN IT BE DELEGATED?

You might think that this is the same question as who can practice medicine, but it is not. This question gets to the issue: what can be delegated, and to whom?

As I explained, a doctor (or an NP or PA in some states) must assess a patient and set a treatment plan. But the doctor can delegate the actual performance of that treatment to someone else. But who can that be? That depends on the state. In some states, it could actually be *anyone*—literally anyone that the doctor decides can do it. In Texas, you can train anyone off the street to inject Botox®, and as long as you (the doc) decide they are trained, it is legal to delegate to them. This is not true in most states. In most states, you have to be at least a licensed RN. But in Texas and a few other states, they leave it up to the physician to decide whom to train. As a consequence, there are many aestheticians out there with no medical training who are injecting.

As we said earlier, you can't go to a spa and be seen by the aesthetician and have injections without a good faith exam by a physician. But after that good faith exam is done and the physician recommends injections, that nurse or other injector may legally carry out the treatment. The rules around delegation are also complicated and different in many states. But you get the idea.

ARRESTS IN TEXAS AND CALIFORNIA

In late 2018, there was a moment when I thought someone was actually going to enforce the law. Four people in Texas were arrested for the illegal practice of medicine. This included a nurse and the doctor who was supposed to be overseeing her and the spa owner of Savvy Chic Medspa in Spring, Texas (which, by the way, in 2024 continues to operate and has a five-star rating on Google). There was a separate arrest of a medical assistant who was illegally injecting unsupervised on her own, in addition to illegally prescribing meds on a stolen prescription pad. The charges against the three involved from the Savvy Chic spa were ultimately dropped. The action against the medical assistant was still pending as of the last information available. I could not find any resolution to that case.

Soon after the Texas arrests, there were two in Redding, California, in January 2019. Susan Ann Tancredo was charged with practicing medicine without a license in addition to eight felony violations, including mayhem, battery with serious bodily injury, and selling and transporting a controlled substance.[21] Dr. Larry Richard Pyle also was charged with aiding and abetting Tancredo.[22] The doctor illegally bought Botox® and other injectables from outside the United States and sold them to Tancredo, who offered illegal injections at a day spa. Patients thought she was a nurse, but she had no medical license. The spa owner was not charged, but then all three were sued by a disfigured patient.

DEATH IN TEXAS

Jennifer Cleveland, a forty-seven-year-old mother of four kids, worked at a radio station in Texas, selling advertising. She was doing some social media marketing for "The Luxe Medspa by Amber Johnson." On July 13, 2023, she told her friends she was going to the spa in

21   Ashley Gardner, "Shasta County Woman in 'Bad Botox' Case Sentenced," KRCRTV.com, March 31, 2023, https://krcrtv.com/news/local/shasta-county-woman-in-bad-botox-case-sentenced.

22   David Benda, "Shasta County DA's Office Says More People Have Come Forward in Illegal Botox Case," Record Searchlight, January 22, 2019, https://www.redding.com/story/news/local/2019/01/22/redding-doctor-botox-case-enters-no-plea-second-court-appearance-shasta-county/2647228002/.

Wortham, Texas, for an IV infusion treatment. She died a few hours later at the spa.

The med spa advertised on its Facebook page: "I (Amber Johnson) am behind this Medspa. I am a Certified Practitioner with all current licenses with a Medical Director, Dr Gallagher MD from Dallas, Texas."

Her spa advertised many procedures that make no sense, such as "Laser Vein Threading" and "Body Extraction—Face." It also advertised three different kinds of IV "therapy," including "energy," "Hydration 1 treatment," and "hydration (three pack)."

First, there is no medical reason a healthy human being needs an IV treatment. There are "IV clinics" popping up all over the country charging you money for something you don't need. Just have a glass of water, Gatorade, or your drink of choice.

Second, there is no quicker way to kill someone than to stick a needle in someone's arm. There are so many ways to do it. Hang the wrong thing—boom you're dead. Put the IV in wrong—boom. A superfast way to die is from an air embolus—that's when a lot of air gets into the IV—air does not mix with blood. It travels to the heart, and the heart can no longer pump blood—and you die. Official reports are that Jennifer died of a potassium overdose in the IV. One thing I can tell you, IV infusions cannot be done by someone who does not know what they are doing!

Hospitals source IV fluids from highly regulated medical supply companies. The IV bags are in proper storage, and every time an IV is hung, the nurse checks your ID badge twice before proceeding. There are tons of checks and balances to try to prevent medical errors. They can still happen.

Med spas, especially those run by nonmedical people, get products from lots of nonmedical sources and have little ability for proper storage and no checks and balances. Plus, who is the person providing the service? Do you know what their credentials are, or what training the person doing the procedure has had?

Dr. Michael Gallagher, the medical director, had his license suspended for a few months, but it was later reinstated and he returned to practicing anesthesiology. The website for this spa has been taken down. The Yelp listing still exists, with a single one-star review:

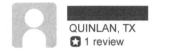

QUINLAN, TX
⭐ 1 review

★☆☆☆☆ 7/14/2023

I don't advise anyone to use your services unless they want to end up dead like my cousin.

WHAT TO ASK BEFORE YOU HAVE A TREATMENT?

- Who owns this spa?
- Who is the medical director? When are they working here?
- Who is doing my good faith exam, and what is their license?
- Who is doing the treatment, and what is their license?

AMSPA, MEDICAL SPA LAW, AND REGULATION

The founder of AmSpa is a lawyer who worked with the med spa industry before starting the association. I joined AmSpa my first year in business and went to the very first annual meeting and have been attending each year since then (even in 2020—it was in January that year). AmSpa has become the de facto association for the medical spa industry. Though there are many aesthetics societies that focus on the practice of aesthetic medicine, AmSpa focuses on the business and legal side as well as the clinical side of the industry.

AmSpa has a stake in making sure that its member spas operate legally. They offer all kinds of advice and many lectures at its various meetings and boot camps. Many med spas do their best to comply with the laws. But compliance is costly. You must set up proper legal structures and financial accounts, and you have to hire those pesky expensive doctors. Many spas cut corners.

Lawyers can help these spas to function legally, on paper. They set up the MSO and arrange the agreements (MSAs) with medical directors. But they can't set up the financial pathways for the spa. Since the money for a medical procedure must go to the doctor first, and then the doctor pays the MSO (spa owner) a management fee, the MSO often gets antsy about that—they want to control the money. But they have to set up the bank account that receives the money under the medical practice name. So to be legal, they would have to give up control of the intake of the money. But they don't do that. They build into the MSA an agreement to manage that bank account for the doctor. This way, they can control the money and hire whatever medical director they can find, for the least amount of money.

The lawyers are really helping to increase compliance but not always to the benefit of the patient. Because in the end, they are often facilitating the nonmedical spa owner to practice medicine, with the minimum involvement possible of an actual doctor.

To AmSpa's credit, they truly believe that adherence to the law is the right thing to do and that legal compliance will benefit consumers and patients in the end. They put together a task force of stakeholders to design a set of legal guidelines for the industry. They published this set of guidelines to their members at the same time as launching an effort in the Texas legislature to introduce these guidelines into law.

There was a massive mutiny among the members. Some members were excited to see the beginnings of self-regulation in the industry. We would like to create a uniform set of laws and standards so that patients know that there are standards that must be met in medical aesthetics. But there was a huge uproar among many spa owners that AmSpa was trying to put them out of business, and many of them left the association. The objections were many, but the main reason in my opinion is that they are not operating legally, and they don't want to be forced to do so. In fact, the costs of operating under the guidelines, some claimed, would put them out of business. Some of us are absorbing that cost already because it is the right thing to do. Those that are not, of course, are at a huge financial advantage.

As a consumer, how do you know who is legit? It can be tough. Make sure you are seeing a doctor (or an NP or PA) when you first visit a new med spa. Ask who owns the spa. Ask who does the services. If you don't see a doctor within fifty miles of the place, take your business elsewhere.

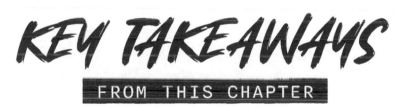

KEY TAKEAWAYS
FROM THIS CHAPTER

1. Ask who owns the medical spa.
2. Who will be doing the good faith exam, and what is their license?
3. Who is the medical director? How often is the medical director working in the spa?
4. Who will be doing the procedure? What is their license?

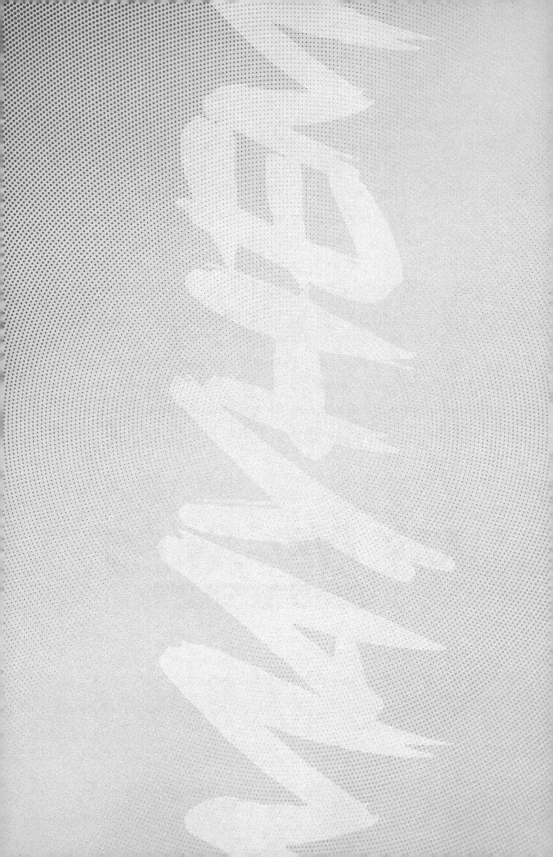

WILL HONESTY AND SCIENCE FINALLY MATTER?

The best consumer is an informed one. I spend so much time with my patients explaining how everything works because I want them to fully understand the science and know that they want to pursue any treatment they might undergo. I talk about science so much not just because I'm a geek (though I am, of course) but also because I truly want to share that knowledge with others. If you truly understand how something works, then you can know if that treatment is right for you. And you'll also understand what to expect, both about the procedure itself and the potential outcomes.

As we have seen in these pages, this is not the norm. The medical aesthetics world is filled with just about everything else, and those of us who rely on science and education are rare zebras in that world. Will our honesty finally matter? I think so. Readers like you will spread the word, and as this information becomes more widespread, and as the aesthetics industry becomes better regulated, I believe there will emerge a better, more reliable, honest and science-based world of medical spas.

Why did I write this book? Many of us in the industry are dumbfounded that there is so much illegal activity in the aesthetics space. I've reached out to attorneys for the city, county, and state. They all say that it is not within their purview until a crime is committed, and even then, it has to be a major crime. Botox® Bandits often get away with it. Bait and Switch is legal. But death and disfigurement—that's where they draw the line. Well, I think that people need to be informed before that happens. Ask the right questions; do your homework. And keep the conversation going.

WEBSITE CONTENT

I hope you will check the website: medspamayhem.com and listen to the podcast "Medspa Mayhem." There you will find updated clinical recommendations mentioned in this book, in addition to online-only topics, including the following. In the podcast, we take a deep dive into everything you've just read and many more topics in the med spa industry.

- Skin Care
- Anti-Aging Ingredients
- Preventive care and maintenance of the skin
- Vitamin D, Sun Block, Sunlight, and Cancer
- Treatments for hair loss
- Body Sculpting
- and more

ACKNOWLEDGMENTS

This book could not have been written without my dad, Thomas J. Dee, who occupies a niche in the back of my brain, advising me as I go through life. Though he didn't live to see the success of my business or the creation of this book, he is an ever-present voice in my life. His sage advice over the years kept me going through the pain and misery of medical education and training, and his keen economic insights have inspired me to make the sound decisions that have allowed my success. Thanks, Dad.

Dr. Carole Stearns, my high school chemistry and physics teacher, gave me advice I didn't particularly want to hear many years ago: to change my career at least once but better yet, twice, or else watch my brain go stale and grow ever more bored. At the time I thought it would never happen. But her words stuck. And as opportunities to change appeared, I embraced the chance. I'm so happy I did. Had it not been for her urging, I may never have tried new things at age forty or even fifty.

To Annika Andrews, thank you for brainstorming with me over lunches and dinners, and encouraging me to take the leap away from Big Medicine.

I am blessed with the absolute best staff anyone could ever ask for. Together, we have navigated the chaos described in these pages and lived to laugh about it all. Thank you, Joanna, Whitney, Toni, Danielle, Fiona, Hannah, Paige, and Kat. And special thanks to Leslie Bratsanos who supported me from day one, knowing this was going to be a thing.

To Sue Petcoff and Lynn Haspedis, thank you for urging me to check out aesthetic medicine. You told me it was "right up my alley" and you were spot on.

To Leslie Baumann, MD, and Yael Halaas, MD: you have both influenced me tremendously as mentors and close friends. Thank you for sharing your stories. And I am so grateful for Naomi Busch, MD for her business acumen, brilliance, and friendship.

To Loren Hosford, the one laser rep who doesn't lie, and has helped Glow become a great success.

To Kathleen Derubeis, who rose in the industry along with me. I couldn't have done it without you!

Thanks to Suzanna de Boer, my editor, who helped shape *Med Spa Mayhem* into something resembling an organized book.

To Felicia Garrett, my best friend and confidant. I don't think I could have survived the last decade without you.

To Ashley Kangas. Thanks, love. Your confidence in me keeps me aloft. Your wisdom keeps me grounded.

To my kids, Zoe, Sierra, and Jason, who have been my biggest cheerleaders. They all worked to make our first open house a success and Zoe was our first Social Media Master, though she might say that's a bit cringy. Sierra connected me to Romy and Michele, the biggest compliment. And for Jason, whose interest in the business side and all the great questions that have helped me clarify my own thinking. They have all put up with my myriad stories and might have told me more than once to "write a book, Mom."

And greatest thanks to every patient who has ever walked through our door. Thank you for believing in me and for being part of the Glow family.

ABOUT THE AUTHOR

DR. KATE DEE grew up in New York City and attended Yale for college and medical school, finishing her MD in 1994. She trained in diagnostic imaging at the University of Washington in Seattle, followed by a fellowship in breast imaging at the University of California, San Francisco, finishing in 2000. She was an assistant professor of medicine at the University of Washington for three years and then a breast cancer specialist at Seattle Breast Center until 2015. Dr. Dee transitioned to aesthetic medicine in her forties, founding Glow Medispa, where she performs all aspects of medical aesthetics from injectables and skin care to lasers and body sculpting. In addition to her medical practice, Dr. Dee has a special interest in business ethics and the medicolegal aspects of practicing aesthetic medicine.

Kate lives in West Seattle and is the proud mom of three amazing kids. She especially loves to ski, cycle, play tennis, and cook.

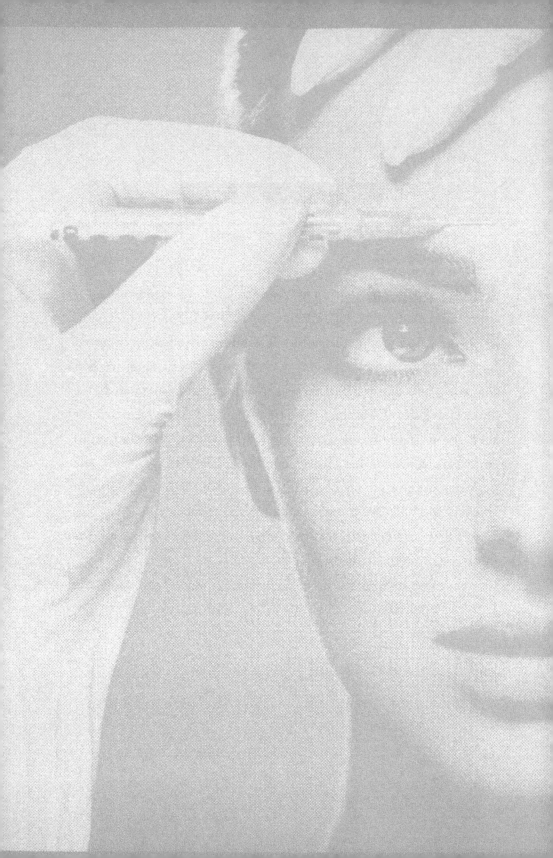

Dr. Kate Dee practices medicine at Glow Medispa in West Seattle:
4409 California Ave SW, Suite 100, Seattle, WA 98116
206-228-7281

Glow Medispa inquiries: info@glowspaseattle.com
www.Glowspaseattle.com
Facebook: glowspaseattle
Instagram: Glow.Medispa

Dr. Dee's website: www.drkatedee.com
Author inquiries: info@drkatedee.com
Facebook: drkatedee
Instagram: drkatedee

Online content for Medspa Mayhem can be found at
www.drkatedee.com or www.medspamayhem.com

Join Dr. Dee on the podcast: Medspa Mayhem